How & When *to be* Your Own Doctor

by

Dr. Isabelle A. Moser *with* Steve Solomon

Table of Contents

Copyright © 2010 Watchmaker Publishing

ISBN 978-1-60386-344-5

Forward

I was a physically tough, happy-go-lucky fellow until I reached my late thirties. Then I began to experience more and more off days when I did not feel quite right. I thought I possessed an iron constitution. Although I grew a big food garden and ate mostly "vegetablitarian" I thought I could eat anything with impunity. I had been fond of drinking beer with my friends while nibbling on salty snacks or heavy foods late into the night. And until my health began to weaken I could still get up the next morning after several homebrewed beers, feeling good, and would put in a solid day's work.

When my health began to slip I went looking for a cure. Up to that time the only use I'd had for doctors was to fix a few traumatic injuries. The only preventative health care I concerned myself with was to take a multivitamin pill during those rare spells when I felt a bit run down and to eat lots of vegetables. So I'd not learned much about alternative health care.

Naturally, my first stop was a local general practitioner/MD. He gave me his usual half-hour get-acquainted checkout and opined that there almost certainly was nothing wrong with me. I suspect I had the good fortune to encounter an honest doctor, because he also said if it were my wish he could send me around for numerous tests but most likely these would not reveal anything either. More than likely, all that was wrong was that I was approaching 40; with the onset of middle age I would naturally have more aches and pains. 'Take some aspirin and get used to it,' was his advice. 'It'll only get worse.'

Not satisfied with his dismal prognosis I asked an energetic old guy I knew named Paul, an '80-something homesteader who was renowned for his organic garden and his good health. Paul referred me to his doctor, Isabelle Moser, who at that time was running the Great Oaks School of Health, a residential and out-patient spa nearby at Creswell, Oregon.

Dr. Moser had very different methods of analysis than the medicos, was warmly personal and seemed very safe to talk to. She looked me over, did some strange magical thing she called muscle testing and concluded that I still had a very strong constitution. If I would eliminate certain "bad" foods from my diet, eliminate some generally healthful foods that, unfortunately, I was allergic to, if I would reduce my alcohol intake greatly and take some food supplements, then gradually my symptoms would abate. With the persistent application of a little self-discipline over several months, maybe six months, I could feel really well again almost all the time and would probably continue that way for many years to come. This was good news, though the need to apply personal responsibility toward the solution of my problem seemed a little sobering.

But I could also see that Dr. Moser was obviously not telling me something. So I gently pressed her for the rest. A little shyly, reluctantly, as though she were used to being rebuffed for making such suggestions, Isabelle asked me if I had ever heard of fasting? "Yes," I said. "I had. Once when I was about twenty and staying at a farm in Missouri, during a bad flu I actually did fast, mainly because I was too sick to take anything but water for nearly one week."

"Why do you ask?" I demanded.

"If you would fast, you will start feeling really good as soon as the fast is over." she said.

"Fast? How long?"

"Some have fasted for a month or even longer," she said. Then she observed my crestfallen expression and added, "Even a couple of weeks would make an enormous difference."

It just so happened that I was in between set-up stages for a new mail-order business I was starting and right then I did have a couple of weeks when I was virtually free of responsibility. I could also face the idea of not eating for a couple of weeks. "Okay!" I said somewhat impulsively. "I could fast for two weeks. If I start right now maybe even three weeks, depending on how my schedule works out."

So in short order I was given several small books about fasting to read at home and was mentally preparing myself for several weeks of severe privation, my only sustenance to be water and herb tea without sweetener. And then came the clinker.

"Have you ever heard of colonics?" she asked sweetly.

"Yes. Weird practice, akin to anal sex or something?"

"Not at all," she responded. "Colonics are essential during fasting or you will have spells when you'll feel terrible. Only colonics make water fasting comfortable and safe."

Then followed some explanation about bowel cleansing (and another little book to take home) and soon I was agreeing to get my body over to her place for a colonic every two or three days during the fasting period, the first colonic scheduled for the next afternoon. I'll spare you a detailed description of my first fast with colonics; you'll read about others shortly. In the end I withstood the boredom of water fasting for 17 days. During the fast I had about 7 colonics. I ended up feeling great, much trimmer, with an enormous rebirth of energy. And when I resumed eating it turned out to be slightly easier to control my dietary habits and appetites.

Thus began my practice of an annual health-building water fast. Once a year, at whatever season it seemed propitious, I'd set aside a couple of weeks to heal my body. While fasting I'd slowly drive myself over to Great Oaks School for colonics every other day. By the end of my third annual fast in 1981, Isabelle and I had become great friends. About this same time Isabelle's relationship with her first husband, Douglas Moser, had disintegrated. Some months later, Isabelle and I became partners. And then we married.

My regular fasts continued through 1984, by which time I had recovered my fundamental organic vigor and had retrained my dietary habits. About 1983 Isabelle and I also began using Life Extension megavitamins as a therapy against the aging process. Feeling so much better I began to find the incredibly boring weeks of prophylactic fasting too difficult to motivate myself to do, and I stopped. Since that time I fast only when acutely ill. Generally less than one week on water handles any non-optimum health condition I've had since '84. I am only 54 years old as I write these words, so I hope it will be many, many years before I find myself in the position where I have to fast for an extended period to deal with a serious or life-threatening condition.

I am a kind of person the Spanish call *autodidactico*, meaning that I prefer to teach myself. I had already learned the fine art of self-employment and general small-business practice that way, as well as radio and electronic theory, typography and graphic design, the garden seed business, horticulture, and agronomy. When Isabelle moved in with me she also brought most of Great Oak's extensive library, including very hard to obtain copies of the works of the early hygienic doctors. Naturally I studied her books intensely.

Isabelle also brought her medical practice into our house. At first it was only a few loyal local clients who continued to consult with her on an out-patient basis, but after a few years, the demands for residential care from people who were seriously and sometimes life-threateningly sick grew irresistibly, and I found myself sharing our family house with a parade of really sick people. True, I was not their doctor, but because her residential clients became temporary parts of our family, I helped support and encourage our residents through their fasting process. I'm a natural teacher (and how-to-do-it writer), so I found myself explaining many aspects of hygienic medicine to Isabelle's clients, while having a first-hand opportunity to observe for myself the healing process at work. Thus it was that I became the doctor's assistant and came to practice second-hand hygienic medicine.

In 1994, when Isabelle had reached the age of 54, she began to think about passing on her life's accumulation of healing wisdom by writing a book. She had no experience at writing for the popular market, her only major writing being a Ph.D. dissertation. I on the other hand had published seven books about vegetable gardening. And I grasped the essentials of her wisdom as well as any non-practitioner could. So we took a summer off and rented a house in rural Costa Rica, where I helped Isabelle put down her thoughts on a cheap word-processing typewriter. When we returned to the States, I fired-up my "big-mac" and composed this manuscript into a rough book format that was given to some of her clients to get what is trendily called these days, "feedback."

But before we could completely finish her book, Isabelle became dangerously ill and after a long, painful struggle with abdominal cancer, she died. After I resurfaced from the worst of my grief and loss, I decided to finish her book. Fortunately, the manuscript needed little more than polishing. I am telling the reader these things because many ghost-written books end up having little direct connection with the originator of the thoughts. Not so in this case. And unlike many ghost writers, I had a long and loving apprenticeship with the author. At every step of our collaboration on this book I have made every effort to communicate Isabelle's viewpoints in the way she would speak, not my own. Dr. Isabelle Moser was for many years my dearest friend. I have worked on this book to help her pass her understanding on.

Many people consider death to be a complete invalidation of a healing arts practitioner. I don't. Coping with her own dicey health had been a major motivator for Isabelle's interest in healing others. She will tell you more about it in the chapters to come. Isabelle had been fending off cancer since its first blow up when she was 26 years old. I view that 30 plus years of defeating Death as a great success rather than consider her ultimate defeat as a failure.

Isabelle Moser was born in 1940 and died in 1996. I think the greatest accomplishment of her 56 years was to meld virtually all available knowledge about health and healing into a workable and most importantly, a simple model that allowed her to have amazing success. Her "system" is simple enough that even a generally well-educated non-medico like me can grasp it. And use it without consulting a doctor every time a symptom appears.

Finally, I should mention that over the years since this book was written I have discovered contains some significant errors of anatomical or physiological detail. Most of these happened because the book was written "off the top of Isabelle's head," without any reference materials at hand, not even an anatomy text. I have not fixed these goofs as I am not even qualified to find them all. Thus, when the reader reads such as 'the pancreas secretes enzymes into the stomach,' (actually and correctly, the duodenum) I hope they will understand and not invalidate the entire book.

Chapter One

How I Became *a* Hygienist

From The Hygienic Dictionary

Doctors. [1] In the matter of disease and healing, the people have been treated as serfs. The doctor is a dictator who knows it all, and the people are stupid, dumb, driven cattle, fit for nothing except to be herded together, bucked and gagged when necessary to force medical opinion down their throats or under their skins. I found that professional dignity was more often pomposity, sordid bigotry and gilded ignorance. The average physician is a fear-monger, if he is anything. He goes about like a roaring lion, seeking whom he may scare to death. *Dr. John. H. Tilden, Impaired Health: Its Cause and Cure, Vol. 1, 1921.* [2] Today we are not only in the Nuclear Age but also the Antibiotic Age. Unhappily, too, this is the Dark Age of Medicine–an age in which many of my colleagues, when confronted with a patient, consult a volume which rivals the Manhattan telephone directory in size. This book contains the names of thousands upon thousands of drugs used to alleviate the distressing symptoms of a host of diseased states of the body. The doctor then decides which pink or purple or baby-blue pill to prescribe for the patient. This is not, in my opinion, the practice of medicine. Far too many of these new "miracle" drugs are introduced with fanfare and then reveled as lethal in character, to be silently discarded for newer and more powerful drugs.
Dr. Henry Bieler: Food is Your Best Medicine; 1965.

I have two reasons for writing this book. One, to help educate the general public about the virtues of natural medicine. The second, to encourage the next generation of natural healers. Especially the second because it is not easy to become a natural hygienist; there is no school or college or licensing board.

Most AMA-affiliated physicians follow predictable career paths, straight well-marked roads, climbing through apprenticeships in established institutions to high financial rewards and social status. Practitioners of natural medicine are not awarded equally high status, rarely do we become wealthy, and often, naturopaths arrive at their profession rather late in life after following the tangled web of their own inner light. So I think it is worth a few pages to explain how I came to practice a dangerous profession and why I have accepted the daily risks of police prosecution and civil liability without possibility of insurance.

Sometimes it seems to me that I began this lifetime powerfully predisposed to heal others. So, just for childhood warm-ups I was born into a family that would be much in need of my help. As I've always disliked an easy win, to make rendering that help even more difficult, I decided to be the youngest child, with two older brothers.

A pair of big, capable brothers might have guided and shielded me. But my life did not work out that way. The younger of my two brothers, three years ahead of me, was born with many health problems. He was weak, small, always ill, and in need of protection from other children, who are generally rough and cruel. My father abandoned our family shortly after I was born; it fell to my mother to work to help support us. Before I was adolescent my older brother left home to pursue a career in the Canadian Air Force.

Though I was the youngest, I was by far the healthiest. Consequently, I had to pretty much raise myself while my single mother struggled to earn a living in rural western Canada. This circumstance probably reinforced my constitutional predilection for independent thought and action. Early on I started to protect my "little" brother, making sure the local bullies didn't take advantage of him. I learned to fight big boys and win. I also helped him acquire simple skills, ones that most kids grasp without difficulty, such as swimming, bike riding, tree climbing, etc.

And though not yet adolescent, I had to function as a responsible adult in our household. Stressed by anger over her situation and the difficulties of earning our living as a country school teacher (usually in remote one-room schools), my mother's health deteriorated rapidly. As she steadily lost energy and became less able to take care of the home, I took over more and more of the cleaning, cooking, and learned how to manage her—a person who feels terrible but must work to survive.

During school hours my mother was able to present a positive attitude, and was truly a gifted teacher. However, she had a personality quirk. She obstinately preferred to help the most able students become even more able, but she had little desire to help those with marginal mentalities. This predilection got her into no end of trouble with local school boards; inevitably it seemed the District Chairman would have a stupid, badly-behaved child that my mother refused to cater to. Several times we had to move in the middle of the school year when she was dismissed without notice for "insubordination." This would inevitably happen on the frigid Canadian Prairies during mid-winter.

At night, exhausted by the day's efforts, my mother's positiveness dissipated and she allowed her mind to drift into negative thoughts, complaining endlessly about my irresponsible father and about how much she disliked him for treating her so badly. These emotions and their irresponsible expression were very difficult for me to deal with as a child, but it taught me to work on diverting someone's negative thoughts, and to avoid getting dragged into them myself, skills I had to use continually much later on when I began to manage mentally and physically ill clients on a residential basis.

My own personal health problems had their genesis long before my own birth. Our diet was awful, with very little fresh fruit or vegetables. We normally had canned, evaporated milk, though there were a few rare times when raw milk and free-range fertile farm eggs were available from neighbors. Most of my foods were heavily salted or sugared, and we ate a great deal of fat in the form of lard. My mother had little money but she had no idea that some of the most nutritious foods are also the least expensive.

It is no surprise to me that considering her nutrient-poor, fat-laden diet and stressful life, my mother eventually developed severe gall bladder problems. Her degeneration caused progressively more and more severe pain until she had a cholecystectomy. The gallbladder's profound deterioration had damaged her liver as well, seeming to her surgeon to require the removal of half her liver. After this surgical insult she had to stop working and never regained her health. Fortunately, by this time all her children were independent.

I had still more to overcome. My eldest brother had a nervous breakdown while working on the DEW Line (he was posted on the Arctic Circle watching radar screens for a possible incoming attack from Russia). I believe his collapse actually began with our childhood nutrition. While in the Arctic all his foods came from cans. He also was working long hours in extremely cramped quarters with no leave for months in a row, never going outside because of the cold, or having the benefit of natural daylight.

When he was still in the acute stage of his illness (I was still a teenager myself) I went to the hospital where my brother was being held, and talked the attending psychiatrist into immediately discharging him into my care. The physician also agreed to refrain from giving him electroshock therapy, a commonly used treatment for mental conditions in Canadian hospitals at that time. Somehow I knew the treatment they were using was wrong.

I brought my brother home still on heavy doses of thorazine. The side effects of this drug were so severe he could barely exist: blurred vision, clenched jaw, trembling hands, and restless feet that could not be kept still. These are common problems with the older generation of psycho tropic medications, generally controlled to some extent with still other drugs like cogentin (which he was taking too).

My brother steadily reduced his tranquilizers until he was able to think and do a few things. On his own he started taking a lot of B vitamins and eating whole grains. I do not know exactly why he did this, but I believe he was following his intuition. (I personally did not know enough to suggest a natural approach at that time.) In any case after three months on vitamins and an improved diet he no long needed any medication, and was delighted to be free of their side effects. He remained somewhat emotionally fragile for a few more months but he soon returned to work, and has had no mental trouble from that time to this day. This was the beginning of my interest in mental illness, and my first exposure to the limitations of 'modern' psychiatry.

I always preferred self-discipline to being directed by others. So I took every advantage of having a teacher for a mother and studied at home instead of being bored silly in a classroom. In Canada of that era you didn't have to go to high school to enter university, you only had to pass the written government entrance exams. At age 16, never having spent a single day in high school, I passed the university entrance exams with a grade of 97 percent. At that point in my life I really wanted to go to medical school and become a doctor, but I didn't have the financial backing to embark on such a long and costly course of study, so I settled on a four year nursing course at the University of Alberta, with all my expenses paid in exchange for work at the university teaching hospital.

At the start of my nurses training I was intensely curious about everything in the hospital: birth, death, surgery, illness, etc. I found most births to be joyful, at least when everything came out all right. Most people died very alone in the hospital, terrified if they were conscious, and all seemed totally unprepared for death, emotionally or spiritually. None of the hospital staff wanted to be with a dying person except me; most hospital staff were unable to confront death any more bravely than those who were dying. So I made it a point of being at the death bed. The doctors and nurses found it extremely unpleasant to have to deal with the preparation of the dead body for the morgue; this chore usually fell to me also. I did not mind dead bodies. They certainly did not mind me!

I had the most difficulty accepting surgery. There were times when surgery was clearly a life saving intervention, particularly when the person had incurred a traumatic injury, but there were many other cases when, though the knife was the treatment of choice, the results were disastrous.

Whenever I think of surgery, my recollections always go to a man with cancer of the larynx. At that time the University of Alberta had the most respected surgeons and cancer specialists in the country. To treat cancer they invariably did surgery, plus radiation and chemotherapy to eradicate all traces of cancerous tissue in the body, but they seemed to forget there also was a human being residing in that very same cancerous body. This particularly unfortunate man came into our hospital as a whole human being, though sick with cancer. He could still speak, eat, swallow, and looked normal. But after surgery he had no larynx, nor esophagus, nor tongue, and no lower jaw.

The head surgeon, who, by the way, was considered to be a virtual god amongst gods, came back from the operating room smiling from ear to ear, announcing proudly that he had 'got all the cancer'. But when I saw the result I thought he'd done a butcher's job. The victim couldn't speak at all, nor eat except through a tube, and he looked grotesque. Worst, he had lost all will to live. I thought the man would have been much better off to keep his body parts as long as he could, and die a whole person able to speak, eating if he felt like it, being with friends and family without inspiring a gasp of horror.

I was sure there must be better ways of dealing with degenerative conditions such as cancer, but I had no idea what they might be or how to find out. There was no literature on medical alternatives in the university library, and no one in the medical school ever hinted at the possibility except when the doctors took jabs at chiropractors. Since no one else viewed the situation as I did I started to think I might be in the wrong profession.

It also bothered me that patients were not respected, were not people; they were considered a "case" or a "condition." I was frequently reprimanded for wasting time talking to patients, trying to get acquainted. The only place in the hospital where human contact was acceptable was the psychiatric ward. So I enjoyed the rotation to psychiatry for that reason, and decided that I would like to make psychiatry or psychology my specialty.

By the time I finished nursing school, it was clear that the hospital was not for me. I especially didn't like its rigid hierarchical system, where all bowed down to the doctors. The very first week in school we were taught that when entering an elevator, make sure that the doctor entered first, then the intern, then the charge nurse. Followed by, in declining order of status: graduate nurses, third year nurses, second year nurses, first year nurses, then nursing aids, then orderlies, then ward clerks, and only then, the cleaning staff. No matter what the doctor said, the nurse was supposed to do it immediately without question–a very military sort of organization.

Nursing school wasn't all bad. I learned how to take care of all kinds of people with every variety of illness. I demonstrated for myself that simple nursing care could support a struggling body through its natural healing process. But the doctor-gods tended to belittle and denigrate nurses. No wonder–so much of nursing care consists of unpleasant chores like bed baths, giving enemas and dealing with other bodily functions.

I also studied the state-of-the-art science concerning every conceivable medical condition, its symptoms, and treatment. At the university hospital nurses were required to take the same pre-med courses as the doctors–including anatomy, physiology, biochemistry, and pharmacology. Consequently, I think it is essential for holistic healers to first ground themselves in the basic sciences of the body's physiological systems. There is also much valuable data in standard medical texts about the digestion, assimilation, and elimination. To really understand illness, the alternative practitioner must be fully aware of the proper functioning of the cardiovascular/pulmonary system, the autonomic and voluntary nervous system, the endocrine system, plus the mechanics and detailed nomenclature of the skeleton, muscles, tendons and ligaments. Also it is helpful to know the conventional medical models for treating various disorders, because they do appear to work well for some people, and should not be totally invalidated simply on the basis of one's philosophical or religious viewpoints.

Many otherwise well-meaning holistic practitioners, lacking an honest grounding in science, sometimes express their understanding of the human body in non-scientific, metaphysical terms that can seem absurd to the well-instructed. I am not denying here that there is a spiritual aspect to health and illness; I believe there are energy flows in and around the body that can effect physiological functioning. I am only suggesting that to discuss illness without hard science is like calling oneself a abstract artist because the painter has no ability to even do a simple, accurate representational drawing of a human figure.

Though hospital life had already become distasteful to me I was young and poor when I graduated. So after nursing school I buckled down and worked just long enough to save enough money to obtain a masters degree in Clinical Psychology from the University of British Columbia. Then I started working at Riverview Hospital in Vancouver, B.C., doing diagnostic testing, and group therapy, mostly with psychotic people. At Riverview I had a three-year-long opportunity to observe the results of conventional psychiatric treatment.

The first thing I noticed was the 'revolving door' phenomena. That is, people go out, and then they're back in, over and over again, demonstrating that standard treatment–drugs, electroshock and group therapy–had been ineffective. Worse, the treatments given at Riverside were dangerous, often with long term side effects that were more damaging than the disease being treated. It felt like nursing school all over again; in the core of my being I somehow knew there was a better way, a more effective way of helping people to regain their mental health. Feeling like an outsider, I started investigating the hospital's nooks and crannies. Much to my surprise, in a back ward, one not open to the public, I noticed a number of people with bright purple skins.

I asked the staff about this and every one of the psychiatrists denied these patients existed. This outright and widely-agreed-upon lie really raised my curiosity. Finally after pouring through the journals in the hospital library I found an article describing psycho tropic-drug-induced disruptions of melanin (the dark skin pigment). Thorazine, a commonly used psychiatric drug, when taken in high doses over a long period of time would do this. Excess melanin eventually was deposited in vital organs such as the heart and the liver, causing death.

I found it especially upsetting to see patients receive electroshock treatments. These violent, physician-induced traumas did seem to disrupt dysfunctional thought patterns such as an impulse to commit suicide, but afterwards the victim couldn't remember huge parts of their life or even recall who they were. Like many other dangerous medical treatments, electroshock can save life but it can also take life away by obliterating identity.

According the Hippocratic Oath, the first criteria of a treatment is that it should do no harm. Once again I found myself trapped in a system that made me feel severe protest. Yet none of these specialists or university professors, or academic libraries had any information about alternatives. Worse, none of these mind-doctor-gods were even looking for better treatments.

Though unpleasant and profoundly disappointing, my experience as a mental hospital psychologist was, like being in nursing school, also very valuable. Not only did I learn how to diagnose, and evaluate the severity of mental illness and assess the dangerousness of the mentally ill, I learned to understand them, to feel comfortable with them, and found that I was never afraid of them. Fearlessness is a huge advantage. The mentally ill seem to have a heightened ability to spot fear in others. If they sense that you are afraid they frequently enjoy terrorizing you. When psychotic people know you feel comfortable with them, and probably understand a great deal of what they are experiencing, when they know that you can and intend to control them, they experience a huge sense of relief. I could always get mentally ill people to tell me what was really going on in their heads when no one else could get them to communicate.

A few years later I married an American and became the Mental Health Coordinator for Whatcom County, the northwestern corner of Washington State. I handled all the legal proceedings in the county for mentally ill people. After treatment in the state mental hospital I supervised their reentry into the community, and attempted to provide some follow up. This work further confirmed my conclusions that in most cases the mentally ill weren't helped by conventional treatment. Most of them rapidly became social problems after discharge. It seemed the mental hospital's only ethically defensible function was incarceration—providing temporary relief for the family and community from the mentally ill person's destructiveness.

I did see a few people recover in the mental health system. Inevitably these were young, and had not yet become institutionalized, a term describing someone who comes to like being in the hospital because confinement feels safe. Hospitalization can mean three square meals and a bed. It frequently means an opportunity to have a sex life (many female inmates are highly promiscuous). Many psychotics are also criminal; the hospital seems far better to them than jail. Many chronically mentally ill are also experts at manipulating the system. When homeless, they deliberately get hospitalized for some outrageous deed just before winter. They then "recover" when the fine weather of spring returns.

After a year as Mental Health Coordinator, I had enough of the "system" and decided that it was as good a time as any to return to school for a Ph.D., this time at University. of Oregon where I studied clinical and counseling psychology and gerontology. While in graduate school I became pregnant and had my first child. Not surprisingly, this experience profoundly changed my consciousness. I realized that it had perhaps been all right for me to be somewhat irresponsible about my own nutrition and health, but that it was not okay to inflict poor nutrition on my unborn child. At that time I was addicted to salty, deep-fat fried corn chips and a diet pop. I thought I had to have these so-called foods every day. I tended to eat for taste, in other words, what I liked, not necessarily what would give me the best nutrition. I was also eating a lot of what most people would consider healthy food: meat, cheese, milk, whole grains, nuts, vegetables, and fruits.

My constitution had seemed strong and vital enough through my twenties to allow this level of dietary irresponsibility. During my early 20s I had even recovered from a breast cancer by sheer will power. (I will discuss this later.) So before my pregnancy I had not questioned my eating habits.

As my body changed and adapted itself to its new purpose I began visiting the libraries and voraciously read everything obtainable under the topic of nutrition–all the texts, current magazines, nutritional journals, and health newsletters. My childhood habit of self-directed study paid off. I discovered alternative health magazines like Let's Live, Prevention, Organic Gardening, and Best Ways, and promptly obtained every back issue since they were first published. Along the way I ran into articles by Linus Pauling on vitamin C, and sent away for all of his books, one of these was co-authored with David Hawkins, called The Orthomolecular Approach to Mental Disorders.

This book had a profound effect on me. I instantly recognized that it was Truth with a capital "T", although the orthomolecular approach was clearly in opposition to the established medical model and contradicted everything I had ever learned as a student or professional. Here at last was the exciting alternative approach to treating mental disorders I had so long sought. I filed this information away, waiting for an opportunity to use it. And I began to study all the references in The Orthomolecular Approach to Mental Disorders dealing with correcting the perceptual functioning of psychotic people using natural substances.

In the course of delving through libraries and book stores, I also came across the Mokelumne Hill Publishing Company (now defunct). This obscure publisher reprinted many unusual and generally crudely reproduced out-of-print books about raw foods diets, hygienic medicine, fruitarianism, fasting, breathairianism, plus some works discussing spiritual aspects of living that were far more esoteric than I had ever thought existed. I decided that weird or not, I might as well find out everything potentially useful. So I spent a lot of money ordering their books. Some of Mokelumne Hill's material really expanded my thoughts. Though much of it seemed totally outrageous, in every book there usually was one line, one paragraph, or if I was lucky one whole chapter that rang true for me.

Recognizing capital "T" Truth when one sees it is one of the most important abilities a person can have. Unfortunately, every aspect of our mass educational system attempts to invalidate this skill. Students are repeatedly told that derivation from recognized authority and/or the scientific method are the only valid means to assess the validity of data. But there is another parallel method to determine the truth or falsehood of information: Knowing. We Know by the simple method of looking at something and recognizing its correctness. It is a spiritual ability. I believe we all have it. But in my case, I never lost the ability to Know because I almost never attended school.

Thus it is that I am absolutely certain How and When to Be Your Own Doctor will be recognized as Truth by some of my readers and rejected as unscientific, unsubstantiated, or anecdotal information by others. I accept this limitation on my ability to teach. If what you read in the following pages seems true for you, great! If it doesn't, there is little or nothing I could do to further convince.

I return now to the time of my first pregnancy. In the face of all these new Truths I was discovering concerning health and nutrition, I made immediate changes in my diet. I severely reduced my animal protein intake and limited cooked food in general. I began taking vitamin and mineral supplements. I also choose a highly atypical Ph.D. dissertation topic, "The Orthomolecular Treatment of Mental Disorders." This fifty cent word, orthomolecular, basically means readjusting the body chemistry by providing unusually large amounts of specific nutrient substances normally found in the human body (vitamins and minerals). Orthomolecular therapy for mental disorders is supported by good diet, by removal of allergy-producing substances, by control of hypoglycemia, plus counseling, and provision of a therapeutic environment.

My proposed dissertation topic met with nothing but opposition. The professors on my doctoral committee had never heard of the word orthomolecular, and all of them were certain it wasn't an accepted, traditional area of research. Research in academia is supposed to be based on the works of a previous researchers who arrived at hypothesis based on data obtained by strictly following scientific methodology. "Scientific" data requires control groups, matched populations, statistical analysis, etc. In my case there was no previous work my dissertation committee would accept, because the available data did not originate from a medical school or psychology department they recognized.

Due to a lot of determination and perseverance I finally did succeed in getting my thesis accepted, and triumphed over my doctoral committee. And I graduated with a dual Ph.D. in both counseling psychology and gerontology. My ambition was to establish the orthomolecular approach on the west coast. At that time I knew of only two clinics in the world actively using nutritional therapy. One was in New York and the other, was a Russian experimental fasting program for schizophrenics. Doctors Hoffer and Osmond had used orthomolecular therapy in a Canadian mental hospital as early as 1950, but they had both gone on to other things.

The newly graduated Dr. Isabelle Moser, Ph.D. was at this point actually an unemployed mother, renting an old, end-of-the-road, far-in-the-country farmhouse; by then I had two small daughters. I strongly preferred to take care of my own children instead of turning them over to a baby sitter. My location and my children made it difficult for me to work any place but at home. So naturally, I made my family home into a hospital for psychotic individuals. I started out with one resident patient at a time, using no psychiatric drugs. I had very good results and learned a tremendous amount with each client, because each one was different and each was my first of each type.

With any psychotic residing in your home it is foolhardy to become inattentive even for one hour, including what are normally considered sleeping hours. I have found the most profoundly ill mentally ill person still to be very crafty and aware even though they may appear to be unconscious or nonresponsive. Psychotics are also generally very intuitive, using faculties most of us use very little or not at all. For example one of my first patients, Christine, believed that I was trying to electrocute her. Though she would not talk, she repeatedly drew pictures depicting this. She had, quite logically within her own reality, decided to kill me with a butcher knife in self-defense before I succeeded in killing her. I had to disarm Christine several times, hide all the household knives, change my sleeping spot frequently, and generally stay sufficiently awake at night to respond to slight, creaky sounds that could indicate the approach of stealthily placed small bare feet.

With orthomolecular treatment Christine improved but also became more difficult to live with as she got better. For example, when she came out of catatonic-like immobility, she became extremely promiscuous, and was determined to sleep with my husband. In fact she kept crawling into bed with him with no clothes on. Either we had to forcefully remove her or the bed would be handed over to her—without a resident man. Christine then decided (logically) that I was an obstacle to her sex life, and once more set out to kill me. This stage also passed, eventually and Christine got tolerably well.

Christine's healing process is quite typical and demonstrates why orthomolecular treatment is not popular. As a psychotic genuinely improves, their aberrated behavior often becomes more aggressive initially and thus, harder to control. It seems far more convenient for all concerned to suppress psychotic behavior with stupefying drugs. A drugged person can be controlled when they're in a sort of perpetual sedation but then, they never get genuinely well, either.

Another early patient, Elizabeth, gave me a particularly valuable lesson, one that changed the direction of my career away from curing insanity and toward regular medicine. Elizabeth was a catatonic schizophrenic who did not speak or move, except for some waxy posturing. She had to be fed, dressed and pottied. Elizabeth was a pretty little brunette who got through a couple of years of college and then spent several years in a state mental hospital. She had recently run away from a hospital, and had been found wandering aimlessly or standing rigidly, apparently staring fixedly at nothing. The emergency mental health facility in a small city nearby called me up and asked if I would take her. I said I would, and drove into town to pick her up. I found Elizabeth in someone's back yard staring at a bush. It took me three hours to persuade her to get in my car, but that effort turned out to be the easiest part of the next months.

Elizabeth would do nothing for herself, including going to the bathroom. I managed to get some nutrition into her, and change her clothes, but that was about all I could do. Eventually she wore me down; I drifted off for an hour's nap instead of watching her all night. Elizabeth slipped away in the autumn darkness and vanished. Needless to say, when daylight came I desperately searched the buildings, the yard, gardens, woods, and even the nearby river. I called in a missing person report and the police looked as well. We stopped searching after a week because there just wasn't any place else to look. Then, into my kitchen, right in front of our round eyes and gaping mouths, walked a smiling, pleasant, talkative young woman who was quite sane.

She said, "Hello I'm Elizabeth! I'm sorry I was such a hassle last week, and thank you for trying to take care of me so well. I was too sick to know any better." She said she had gone out our back door the week before and crawled under a pile of fallen leaves on the ground in our back yard with a black tarp over them. We had looked under the tarp at least fifty times during the days past, but never thought to look under the leaves as well.

This amazing occurrence made my head go bong to say the least; it was obvious that Elizabeth had not been 'schizophrenic' because of her genetics, nor because of stress, nor malnutrition, nor hypoglycemia, nor because of any of the causes of mental illness I had previously learned to identify and rectify, but because of food allergies. Elizabeth was spontaneously cured because she'd had nothing to eat for a week. The composting pile of leaves hiding her had produced enough heat to keep her warm at night and the heap contained sufficient moisture to keep her from getting too dehydrated. She looked wonderful, with clear shiny blue eyes, clear skin with good color, though she was slightly slimmer than when I had last seen her.

I then administered Coca's Pulse Test (see the Appendix) and quickly discovered Elizabeth was wildly intolerant to wheat and dairy products. Following the well known health gurus of that time like Adelle Davis, I had self-righteously been feeding her home-made whole wheat bread from hand-ground Organic wheat, and home-made cultured yogurt from our own organically-fed goats. But by doing this I had only maintained her insanity. Elizabeth was an intelligent young woman, and once she understood what was causing her problems, she had no trouble completely eliminating certain foods from her diet. She shuddered at the thought that had she not come to my place and discovered the problem, she would probably have died on the back ward of some institution for the chronically mentally ill.

As for me, I will always be grateful to her for opening my eyes and mind a little wider. Elizabeth's case showed me why Russian schizophrenics put on a 30 day water fast had such a high recovery rate. I also remembered all the esoteric books I had read extolling the benefits of fasting. I also remembered two occasions during my own youth when I had eaten little or nothing for approximately a month each without realizing that I was "fasting." And doing this had done me nothing but good.

Once when I was thirteen my mother sent my "little" brother and I to a residential fundamentalist bible school. I did not want to go there, although my brother did; he had decided he wanted to be a evangelical minister. I hated bible school because I was allowed absolutely no independence of action. We were required to attend church services three times a day during the week, and five services on Sunday. As I became more and more unhappy, I ate less and less; in short order I wasn't eating at all. The school administration became concerned after I had dropped about 30 pounds in two months, notified my mother and sent me home. I returned to at-home schooling. I also resumed eating.

I fasted one other time for about a month when I was 21. It happened because I had nothing to do while visiting my mother before returning to University except help with housework and prepare meals. The food available in the backwoods of central B.C. didn't appeal to me because it was mostly canned vegetables, canned milk, canned moose meat and bear meat stews with lots of gravy and greasy potatoes. I decided to pass on it altogether. I remember rather enjoying that time as a fine rest and I left feeling very good ready to take on the world full force ahead. At that time I didn't know there was such a thing as fasting, it just happened that way.

After Elizabeth went on her way, I decided to experimentally fast myself. I consumed only water for two weeks. But I must have had counter intentions to this fast because I found myself frequently having dreams about sugared plums, and egg omelets, etc. And I didn't end up feeling much better after this fast was over (although I didn't feel any worse either), because I foolishly broke the fast with one of my dream omelets. And I knew better! Every book I'd ever read on fasting stated how important it is to break a fast gradually, eating only easy-to-digest foods for days or weeks before resuming one's regular diet.

From this experiment I painfully learned how important it is to break a fast properly. Those eggs just didn't feel right, like I had an indigestible stone in my belly. I felt very tired after the omelet, not energized one bit by the food. I immediately cut back my intake to raw fruits and vegetables while the eggs cleared out of my system. After a few days on raw food I felt okay, but I never did regain the shine I had achieved just before I resumed eating.

This is one of the many fine things about fasting, it allows you to get in much better communication with your own body, so that you can hear it when it objects to something you're putting in it or doing to it. It is not easy to acquire this degree of sensitivity to your body unless you remove all food for a sufficiently long period; this allows the body to get a word in edgewise that we are willing and able to listen to. Even when we do hear the body protesting, we frequently decide to turn a deaf ear, at least until the body starts producing severe pain or some other symptom that we can't ignore.

Within a few years after Elizabeth's cure I had handily repaired quite a few mentally ill people in a harmless way no one had heard of; many new people were knocking at my door wanting to be admitted to my drug free, home-based treatment program. So many in fact that my ability to accommodate them was overwhelmed. I decided that it was necessary to move to a larger facility and we bought an old, somewhat run-down estate that I called Great Oaks School of Health because of the magnificent oak trees growing in the front yard.

At Great Oaks initially I continued working with psychotics, employing fasting as a tool, especially in those cases with obvious food allergies as identified by Coca's Pulse Test, because it only takes five days for a fasting body to eliminate all traces of an allergic food substance and return to normal functioning. If the person was so severely hypoglycemic that they were unable to tolerate a water fast, an elimination diet (to be described in detail later) was employed, while stringently avoiding all foods usually found to be allergy producing.

I also decided that if I was going to employ fasting as my primary medicine, it was important for me to have a more intense personal experience with it, because in the process of reviewing the literature on fasting I saw that there were many different approaches, each one staunchly defended by highly partisan advocates. For example, the capital "N" Natural, capital "H" Hygienists, such a Herbert Shelton, aggressively assert that only a pure water fast can be called a fast. Sheltonites contend that juice fasting as advocated by Paavo Airola, for example, is not a fast but rather a modified diet without the benefits of real fasting. Colon cleansing was another area of profound disagreement among the authorities. Shelton strongly insisted that enemas and colonics should not be employed; the juice advocates tend to strongly recommend intestinal cleansing.

To be able to intelligently take a position in this maze of conflict I decided to first try every system on myself. It seems to me that if I can be said to really own anything in this life it is my own body, and I have the absolute right to experiment with it as long as I'm not irresponsible about important things such as care of my kids. I also feel strongly that it was unethical to ask anyone to do anything that I was not willing or able to do myself. Just imagine what would happen if all medical doctors applied this principal in their practice of medicine, if all surgeons did it too!

I set out to do a complete and fully rigorous water fast according to the Natural Hygiene model—only pure water and bed rest (with no colon cleansing) until hunger returns, something the hygienists all assured me would happen when the body had completed its detoxification process. The only aspect of a hygienic fast I could not fulfill properly was the bed rest part; unfortunately I was in sole charge of a busy holistic treatment center (and two little girls); there were things I had to do, though I did my chores and duties at a very slow pace with many rest periods.

I water fasted for 42 days dropping from 135 pounds to 85 pounds on a 5' 7" frame. At the end I looked like a Nazi concentration camp victim. I tended to hide when people came to the door, because the sight of all my bones scared them to death. Despite my assurances visitors assumed I was trying to commit suicide. In any case I persevered, watching my body change, observing my emotions, my mental functioning, and my spiritual awareness. I thought, if Moses could fast for 42 days so can I, even though the average length of a full water fast to skeletal weight for a person that is not overweight is more in the order of 30 days. I broke the fast with small amounts of carrot juice diluted 50/50 with water and stayed on that regimen for two more weeks.

After I resumed eating solid food it took six weeks to regain enough strength to be able to run the same distance in the same time I had before fasting, and it took me about six months to regain my previous weight. My eyes and skin had become exceptionally clear, and some damaged areas of my body such as my twice-broken shoulder had undergone considerable healing. I ate far smaller meals after the fast, but food was so much more efficiently absorbed that I got a lot more miles to the gallon from what I did eat. I also became more aware when my body did not want me to eat something. After the fast, if I ignored my body's protest and persisted, it would immediately create some unpleasant sensation that quickly persuaded me to curb my appetite.

I later experimented with other approaches to fasting, with juice fasts, with colon cleansing, and began to establish my own eclectic approach to fasting and detoxification, using different types of programs for different conditions and adjusting for psychological tolerances. I'll have a lot more to say about fasting.

After my own rigorous fasting experience I felt capable of supervising extended fasts on very ill or very overweight people. Great Oaks was gradually shifting from being a place that mentally ill people came to regain their sanity to being a spa where anyone who wanted to improve their health could come for a few days, some weeks or even a few months. It had been my observation from the beginning that the mentally ill people in my program also improved remarkably in physical health; it was obvious that my method was good for anyone. Even people with good health could feel better.

By this time I'd also had enough of psychotic people anyway, and longed for sane, responsible company.

So people started to come to Great Oaks School of Health to rest up from a demanding job, to drop some excess weight, and generally to eliminate the adverse effects of destructive living and eating habits. I also began to get cancer patients, ranging from those who had just been diagnosed and did not wish to go the AMA-approved medical route of surgery, chemotherapy, and radiation, to those with well-advanced cancer who had been sent home to die after receiving all of the above treatments and were now ready to give alternative therapies a try since they expected to die anyway. I also had a few people who were beyond help because their vital organs had been so badly damaged that they knew they were dying, and they wanted to die in peace without medical intervention, in a supportive hospice cared for by people who could confront death.

Great Oaks School was intentionally named a "school" of health partially to deflect the attentions of the AMA. It is, after all, entirely legal to teach about how to maintain health, about how to prevent illness, and how to go about making yourself well once you were sick. Education could not be called "practicing medicine without a license." Great Oaks was also structured as a school because I wanted to both learn and teach. Toward this end we started putting out a holistic health newsletter and offering classes and seminars to the public on various aspects of holistic health. From the early 1970s through the early 1980s I invited a succession of holistic specialists to reside at GOSH, or to teach at Great Oaks while living elsewhere. These teachers not only provided a service to the community, but they all became my teachers as well. I apprenticed myself to each one in turn.

There came and went a steady parade of alternative practitioners of the healing arts and assorted forms of metapsychology: acupuncturists, acupressurists, reflexologists, polarity therapists, massage therapists, postural integrationists, Rolfers, Feldenkries therapists, neurolinguistic programmers, biokinesiologists, iridologists, psychic healers, laying on of handsers, past life readers, crystal therapists, toning therapists in the person of Patricia Sun, color therapy with lamps and different colored lenses a la Stanley Bourroughs, Bach Flower therapists, aroma therapists, herbalists, homeopaths, Tai Chi classes, yoga classes, Arica classes, Guergieff and Ouspensky fourth-way study groups, EST workshops, Zen Meditation classes. Refugee Lamas from Tibet gave lectures on The Book of the Dead and led meditation and chanting sessions, and we held communication classes using Scientology techniques. There were anatomy and physiology classes, classes on nutrition and the orthomolecular approach to treating mental disorders (given by me of course); there were chiropractors teaching adjustment techniques, even first aid classes. And we even had a few medical doctors of the alternative ilk who were interested in life style changes as an approach to maintaining health.

Classes were also offered on colon health including herbs, clays, enemas, and colonics. So many of my client at Great Oaks were demanding colonics in conjunction with their cleansing programs, that I took time out to go to Indio, Calif. to take a course in colon therapy from a chiropractor, and purchase a state of the art colonic machine featuring all the gauges, electric water solenoids and stainless steel knobs one could ask for.

During this period almost all alternative therapists and their specialties were very interesting to me, but I found that most of the approaches they advocated did not suit my personality. For example, I think that acupuncture is a very useful tool, but I personally did not want to use needles. Similarly I thought that Rolfing was a very effective tool but I did not enjoy administering that much pain, although a significant number of the clients really wanted pain. Some of the techniques appealed to me in the beginning, and I used them frequently with good results but over time I decided to abandon them, mostly because of a desire to simplify and lighten up my bag of tricks.

Because of my enthusiasm and successes Great Oaks kept on growing. Originally the estate served as both the offices of the Holt Adoption Agency and the Holt family mansion. The Holt family had consisted of Harry and Bertha Holt, six of their biological children, and eight adopted Korean orphans. For this reason the ten thousand square foot two story house had large common rooms, and lots and lots of bedrooms. It was ideal for housing spa clients and my own family. The adjoining Holt Adoption Agency office building was also very large with a multitude of rooms. It became living space for those helpers and hangers-on we came to refer to as "community members." My first husband added even more to the physical plant constructing a large, rustic gym and workshop.

Many "alternative" people visited and then begged to stay on with room and board provided in exchange for their work. A few of these people made a significant contribution such as cooking, child care, gardening, tending the ever-ravenous wood-fired boiler we used to keep the huge concrete mansion heated, or doing general cleaning. But the majority of the 'work exchangers' did not really understand what work really was, or didn't have sufficient ethical presence to uphold the principle of fair exchange, which is basically giving something of equal value for getting something of value and, perhaps more importantly, giving in exchange what is needed and asked for.

I also found that community members, once in residence, were very difficult to dislodge. My healing services were supporting far too much dead wood. This was basically my own fault, my own poor management.

Still, I learned a great deal from all of this waste. First of all it is not a genuine service to another human being to give them something for nothing. If a fair exchange is expected and received, positive ethical behavior is strengthened, allowing the individual to maintain their self-respect. I also came to realize what an important factor conducting one's life ethically is in the individual healing process. Those patients who were out exchange in their relationships with others in one or more areas of their life frequently did not get well until they changed these behaviors.

Toward the end of 1982, after providing a decade of services to a great many clients, many of these in critical condition, I reached to point where I was physically, mentally, and spiritually drained. I needed a vacation desperately but no one, including my first husband, could run Great Oaks in my absence much less cover the heavy mortgage. So I decided to sell it. This decision stunned the community members and shocked the clientele who had become dependent on my services. I also got a divorce at this time. In fact I went through quite a dramatic life change in many areas–true to pattern, a classic mid-life crisis. All I kept from these years was my two daughters, my life experiences, and far too many books from the enormous Great Oaks library.

These changes were however, necessary for my survival. Any person who works with, yes, lives on a day-to-day basis with sick people and who is constantly giving or outflowing must take time out to refill their vessel so that they can give again. Failure to do this can result in a serious loss of health, or death. Most healers are empathic people who feel other peoples' pains and stresses and sometimes have difficulty determining exactly what is their own personal 'baggage' and what belongs to the clients. This is especially difficult when the therapy involves a lot of 'hands on' techniques.

After leaving Great Oaks it took me a couple of years to rest up enough to want to resume practicing again. This time, instead of creating a substantial institution, Steve, my second husband and my best friend, built a tiny office next to our family home. I had a guest room that I would use for occasional residential patients. Usually these were people I had known from Great Oaks days or were people I particularly liked and wanted to help through a life crisis.

At the time I am writing this book over ten years have passed since I sold Great Oaks. I continue to have an active outpatient practice, preferring to protect the privacy of my home and family life since I was remarried by limiting inpatients to a special few who required more intensive care, and then, only one at a time, and then, with long spells without a resident.

Chapter Two

The Nature & Cause *of* Disease

From The Hygienic Dictionary

Toxemia. [1] "Toxemia is the basic cause of all so-called diseases. In the process of tissue-building (metabolism), there is cell-building (anabolism) and cell destruction (catabolism). The broken-down tissue is toxic. In the healthy body (when nerve energy is normal), this toxic material is eliminated from the blood as fast as it is evolved. But when nerve energy is dissipated from any cause (such as physical or mental excitement or bad habits) the body becomes weakened or enervated. When the body is enervated, elimination is checked. This, in turn, results in a retention of toxins in the blood–the condition which we speak of as toxemia. This state produces a crisis which is nothing more than heroic or extraordinary efforts by the body to eliminate waste or toxin from the blood. It is this crisis which we term disease. Such accumulation of toxin when once established, will continue until nerve energy has been restored to normal by removing the cause. So-called disease is nature's effort to eliminate toxin from the blood. All so-called diseases are crises of toxemia." *John H. Tilden, M.D., Toxemia Explained.* [2] Toxins are divided into two groups; namely exogenous, those formed in the alimentary canal from fermentation and decomposition following imperfect or faulty digestion. If the fermentation is of vegetables or fruit, the toxins are irritating, stimulating and enervating, but not so dangerous or destructive to organic life as putrefaction, which is a fermentation set up in nitrogenous matter–protein-bearing foods, but particularly animal foods. Endogenous toxins are autogenerated. They are the waste products of metabolism. *Dr. John. H. Tilden, Impaired Health: Its Cause and Cure, 1921.*

Suppose a fast-growing city is having traffic jams. "We don't like it!" protest the voters. "Why are these problems happening?" asks the city council, trying to look like they are doing something about it.

Experts then proffer answers. "Because there are too many cars," says the Get A Horse Society. The auto makers suggest it is because there are uncoordinated traffic lights and because almost all the businesses send their employees home at the same time. Easy to fix! And no reason whatsoever to limit the number of cars. The asphalt industry suggests it is because the size and amount of roads is inadequate.

What do we do then? Tax cars severely until few can afford them? Legislate opening and closing hours of businesses to stagger to'ing and fro'ing? Hire a smarter municipal highway engineer to synchronize the traffic lights? Build larger and more efficient streets? Demand that auto companies make cars smaller so more can fit the existing roads? Tax gasoline prohibitively, pass out and give away free bicycles in virtually unlimited quantities while simultaneously building mass rail systems? What? Which?

When we settle on a solution we have simultaneously chosen what we consider the real, underlying cause of the problem. If our chosen reason was the real reason. then our solution results in a real cure. If we picked wrongly, our attempt at solution may result in no cure, or create a worse situation than we had before.

The American Medical Association style of medicine (a philosophy I will henceforth call allopathic) has a model that explains the causes of illness. It suggests that anyone who is sick is a victim. Either they were attacked by a "bad" organism–virus, bacteria, yeast, pollen, cancer cell, etc.–or they have a "bad" organ–liver, kidney, gall bladder, even brain. Or, the victim may also have been cursed by bad genes. In any case, the cause of the disease is not the person and the person is neither responsible for creating their own complaint nor is the victim capable of making it go away. This institutionalized irresponsibility seems useful for both parties to the illness, doctor and patient. The patient is not required to do anything about their complaint except pay (a lot) and obediently follow the instructions of the doctor, submitting unquestioningly to their drugs and surgeries. The physician then acquires a role of being considered vital to the survival of others and thus obtains great status, prestige, authority, and financial remuneration.

Perhaps because the sick person is seen to have been victimized, and it is logically impossible to consider a victimizer as anything but something evil, the physician's cure is often violent, confrontational. Powerful poisons are used to rejigger body chemistry or to arrest the multiplication of disease bacteria or to suppress symptoms; if it is possible to sustain life without them, "bad," poorly-functioning organs are cut out.

I've had a lot of trouble with the medical profession. Over the years doctors have made attempts to put me in jail and keep me in fear. But they never stopped me. When I've had a client die there has been an almost inevitable coroner's investigation, complete with detectives and the sheriff. Fortunately, I practice in rural Oregon, where the local people have a deeply-held belief in individual liberty and where the authorities know they would have had a very hard time finding a jury to convict me. Had I chosen to practice with a high profile and had I located Great Oaks School of Health in a major market area where the physicians were able to charge top dollar, I probably would have spent years behind bars as did other heroes of my profession such as Linda Hazzard and Royal Lee.

So I have acquired an uncomplimentary attitude about medical doctors, a viewpoint I am going to share with you ungently, despite the fact that doing so will alienate some of my readers. But I do so because most Americans are entirely enthralled by doctors, and this doctor-god worship kills a lot of them.

However, before I get started on the medicos, let me state that one area exists where I do have fundamental admiration for allopathic medicine. This is its handling of trauma. I agree that a body can become the genuine victim of fast moving bullets. It can be innocently cut, smashed, burned, crushed and broken. Trauma are not diseases and modern medicine has become quite skilled at putting traumatized bodies back together. Genetic abnormality may be another undesirable physical condition that is beyond the purview of natural medicine. However, the expression of contra-survival genetics can often be controlled by nutrition. And the expression of poor genetics often results from poor nutrition, and thus is similar to a degenerative disease condition, and thus is well within the scope of natural medicine.

Today's suffering American public is firmly in the AMA's grip. People have been effectively prevented from learning much about medical alternatives, have been virtually brainwashed by clever media management that portrays other medical models as dangerous and/or ineffective. Legislation influenced by the allopathic doctors' union, the American Medical Association, severely limits or prohibits the practice of holistic health. People are repeatedly directed by those with authority to an allopathic doctor whenever they have a health problem, question or confusion. Other types of healers are considered to be at best harmless as long as they confine themselves to minor complaints; at worst, when naturopaths, hygienists, or homeopaths seek to treat serious disease conditions they are called quacks, accused of unlicensed practice of medicine and if they persist or develop a broad, successful, high-profile and (this is the very worst) profitable practice, they are frequently jailed.

Even licensed MDs are crushed by the authorities if they offer non-standard treatments. So when anyone seeks an alternative health approach it is usually because their complaint has already failed to vanish after consulting a whole series of allopathic doctors. This highly unfortunate kind of sufferer not only has a degenerative condition to rectify, they may have been further damaged by harsh medical treatments and additionally, they have a considerable amount of brainwashing to overcome.

The AMA has succeeded at making their influence over information and media so pervasive that most people do not even realize that the doctors' union is the source of their medical outlook. Whenever an American complains of some malady, a concerned and honestly caring friend will demand to know have they yet consulted a medical doctor. Failure to do so on one's own behalf is considered highly irresponsible. Concerned relatives of seriously ill adults who decline standard medical therapy may, with a great show of self-righteousness, have the sick person judged mentally incompetent so that treatment can be forced upon them. When a parent fails to seek standard medical treatment for their child, the adult may well be found guilty of criminal negligence, raising the interesting issue of who "owns" the child, the parents or the State.

It is perfectly acceptable to die while under conventional medical care. Happens all the time, in fact. But holistic alternatives are represented as stupidly risky, especially for serious conditions such as cancer. People with cancer see no choice but to do chemotherapy, radiation, and radical surgery because this is the current allopathic medical approach. On some level people may know that these remedies are highly dangerous but they have been told by their attending oncologist that violent therapies are their only hope of survival, however poor that may be. If a cancer victim doesn't proceed immediately with such treatment their official prognosis becomes worse by the hour. Such scare tactics are common amongst the medical profession, and they leave the recipient so terrified that they meekly and obediently give up all self-determinism, sign the liability waiver, and submit, no questions asked. Many then die after suffering intensely from the therapy, long before the so-called disease could have actually caused their demise. I will later offer alternative and frequently successful (but not guaranteed) approaches to treating cancer that do not require the earliest-possible detection, surgery or poisons.

If holistic practitioners were to apply painful treatments like allopaths use, ones with such poor statistical outcomes like allopaths use, there would most certainly be witch hunts and all such irresponsible, greedy quacks would be safely imprisoned. I find it highly ironic that for at least the past twenty five hundred years the basic principle of good medicine has been that the treatment must first do no harm. This is such an obvious truism that even the AMA doctors pledge to do the same thing when they take the Hippocratic Oath. Yet virtually every action taken by the allopath is a conscious compromise between the potential harm of the therapy and its potential benefit.

In absolute contrast, if a person dies while on a natural hygiene program, they died because their end was inevitable no matter what therapy was attempted. Almost certainly receiving hygienic therapy contributed to making their last days far more comfortable and relatively freer of pain without using opiates. I have personally taken on clients sent home to die after they had suffered everything the doctors could do to them, told they had only a few days, weeks, or months to live. Some of these clients survived as a result of hygienic programs even at that late date. And some didn't. The amazing thing was that any of them survived at all, because the best time to begin a hygienic program is as early in the degenerative process as possible, not after the body has been drastically weakened by invasive and toxic treatments. Later on, I'll tell you about some of these cases.

Something I consider especially ironic is that when the patient of a medical doctor dies, it is inevitably thought that the blessed doctor did all that could be done; rarely is any blame laid. If the physician was especially careless or stupid, their fault can only result in a civil suit, covered by malpractice insurance. But let a holistic practitioner treat a sick person and have that person follow any of their suggestions or take any natural remedies and have that person die or worsen and it instantly becomes the natural doctor's fault. Great blame is placed and the practitioner faces inquests, grand juries, manslaughter charges, jail time and civil suits that can't be insured against.

Allopathic medicine rarely makes a connection between the real causes of a degenerative or infectious disease and its cure. The causes are usually considered mysterious: we don't know why the pancreas is acting up, etc. The sick are sympathized with as victims who did nothing to contribute to their condition. The cure is a highly technical battle against the illness, whose weapons are defined in Latin and far beyond the understanding of a layperson.

Hygienic medicine presents an opposite view. To the naturopath, illness is not a perplexing and mysterious occurrence over which you have no control or understanding. The causes of disease are clear and simple, the sick person is rarely a victim of circumstance and the cure is obvious and within the competence of a moderately intelligent sick person themselves to understand and help administer. In natural medicine, disease is a part of living that you are responsible for, and quite capable of handling.

Asserting that the sick are pitiable victims is financially beneficial to doctors. It makes medical intervention seem a vital necessity for every ache and pain. It makes the sick become dependent. I'm not implying that most doctors knowingly are conniving extortionists. Actually most medical doctors are genuinely well-intentioned. I've also noticed that most medical doctors are at heart very timid individuals who consider that possession of a MD degree and license proves that they are very important, proves them to be highly intelligent, even makes them fully qualified to pontificate on many subjects not related to medicine at all.

Doctors obtain an enormous sense of self-importance at medical school, where they proudly endured the high pressure weeding out of any free spirit unwilling to grind away into the night for seven or more years. Anyone incapable of absorbing and regurgitating huge amounts of rote information; anyone with a disrespectful or irreverent attitude toward the senior doctor-gods who arrogantly serve as med school professors, anyone like this was eliminated with especial rapidity. When the thoroughly submissive, homogenized survivors are finally licensed, they assume the status of junior doctor-gods.

But becoming an official medical deity doesn't permit one to create their own methods. No no, the AMA's professional oversight and control system makes continued possession of the license to practice (and the high income that usually comes with it) entirely dependent on continued conformity to what is defined by the AMA as "correct practice." Any doctor who innovates beyond s   es non-standard treatments is in real danger of losing their livelihood and o.

Not only are licensed graduates of AMA-sanctioned   kept on a very tight leash, doctors of other persuasions who use other r   he sick or help them heal themselves are persecuted and prosecuted. E   AMA's control through regulatory law and police power is justified in th   ating quackery and making sure the ignorant and gullible public receiv   fically proven effective medical care.

Those on the other side of the fence view the AMA's oppression as an effective way to make sure the public has no real choices but to use union doctors, pay their high fees and suffer greatly by misunderstanding of the true cause of disease and its proper cure. If there are any actual villains responsible for this suppressive tragedy some of them are to be found in the inner core of the AMA, officials who may perhaps fully and consciously comprehend the suppressive system they promulgate.

Hygienists usually inform the patient quite clearly and directly that the practitioner has no ability to heal them or cure their condition and that no doctor of any type actually is able to heal. Only the body can heal itself, something it is eager and usually very able to do if only given the chance. One pithy old saying among hygienists goes, "if the body can't heal itself, nothing can heal it." The primary job of the hygienic practitioner is to reeducate the patient by conducting them through their first natural healing process. If this is done well the sick person learns how to get out of their own body's way and permit its native healing power to manifest. Unless later the victim of severe traumatic injury, never again will that person need obscenely expensive medical procedures. Hygienists rarely make six figure incomes from regular, repeat business.

This aspect of hygienic medicine makes it different than almost all the others, even most other holistic methods. Hygiene is the only system that does not interpose the assumed healing power of a doctor between the patient and wellness. When I was younger and less experienced I thought that the main reason traditional medical practice did not stress the body's own healing power and represented the doctor as a necessary intervention was for profit. But after practicing for over twenty years I now understand that the last thing most people want to hear is that their own habits, especially their eating patterns and food choices, are responsible for their disease and that their cure is to only be accomplished through dietary reform, which means unremittingly applied self-discipline.

One of the hardest things to ask of a person is to change a habit. The reason that AMA doctors have most of the patients is they're giving the patients exactly what they want, which is to be allowed to continue in their unconscious irresponsibility.

The Cause *of* Disease

Ever since natural medicine arose in opposition to the violence of so-called scientific medicine, every book on the subject of hygiene, once it gets past its obligatory introductions and warm ups, must address The Cause of Disease. This is a required step because we see the cause of disease and its consequent cure in a very different manner than the allopath. Instead of many causes, we see one basic reason why. Instead of many unrelated cures, we have basically one approach to fix all ills that can be fixed.

A beautiful fifty cent word that means a system for explaining something is paradigm, pronounced para-dime. I am fond of this word because it admits the possibility of many differing yet equally true explanations for the same reality. Of all available paradigms, Natural Hygiene suits me best and has been the one I've used for most of my career.

The Natural Hygienist's paradigm for the cause of both degenerative and infectious disease is called the Theory of Toxemia, or "self-poisoning."

Before explaining this theory it will help many readers if I digress a brief moment about the nature and validity of alternative paradigms. Not too many decades ago, scientists thought that reality was a singular, real, perpetual–that Natural Law existed much as a tree or a rock existed. In physics, for example, the mechanics of Newton were considered capital "T" True, the only possible paradigm. Any other view, not being True, was False. There was capital "N" natural capital "L" law.

More recently, great uncertainty has entered science; it has become indisputable that a theory or explanation of reality is only true only to the degree it seems to work; conflicting or various explanations can all work, all can be "true." At least, this uncertainty has overtaken the hard, physical sciences. It has not yet done so with medicine. The AMA is convinced (or is working hard to convince everyone else) that its paradigm, the allopathic approach, is Truth, is scientific, and therefore, anything else is Falsehood, is irresponsibility, is a crime against the sick.

But the actual worth or truth of any paradigm is found not in its "reality," but in its utility. Does an explanation or theory allow a person to manipulate experience and create a desired outcome. To the extent a paradigm does that, it can be considered valuable. Judged by this standard, the Theory of Toxemia must be far truer than the hodgepodge of psuedoscience taught in medical schools. Keep that in mind the next time some officious medical doctor disdainfully informs you that Theory of Toxemia was disproven in 1927 by Doctors Jeckel and Hyde.

Why People Get Sick

This is the Theory of Toxemia. A healthy body struggles continually to purify itself of poisons that are inevitably produced while going about its business of digesting food, moving about, and repairing itself. The body is a marvelous creation, a carbon, oxygen combustion machine, constantly burning fuel, disposing of the waste products of combustion, and constantly rebuilding tissue by replacing worn out, dead cells with new, fresh ones. Every seven years virtually every cell in the body is replaced, some types of cells having a faster turnover rate than others, which means that over a seven year period several hundred pounds of dead cells must be digested (autolyzed) and eliminated. All by itself this would be a lot of waste disposal for the body to handle. Added to that waste load are numerous mild poisons created during proper digestion. And added to that can be an enormous burden of waste products created as the body's attempts to digest the indigestible, or those tasty items I've heard called "fun food." Add to that burden the ruinous effects of just plain overeating.

The waste products of digestion, of indigestion, of cellular breakdown and the general metabolism are all poisonous to one degree or another. Another word for this is toxic. If these toxins were allowed to remain and accumulate in the body, it would poison itself and die in agony. So the body has a processing system to eliminate toxins. And when that system does break down the body does die in agony, as from liver or kidney failure.

The organs of detoxification remove things from the body's system, but these two vital organs should not be confused with what hygienists call the secondary organs of elimination, such as the large intestine, lungs, bladder and the skin, because none of these other eliminatory organs are supposed to purify the body of toxins. But when the body is faced with toxemia, the secondary organs of elimination are frequently pressed into this duty and the consequences are the symptoms we call illness.

The lungs are supposed to eliminate only carbon dioxide gas; not self-generated toxic substances. The large intestine is supposed to pass only insoluble food solids (and some nasty stuff dumped into the small intestine by the liver). Skin eliminates in the form of sweat (which contains mineral salts) to cool the body, but the skin is not supposed to move toxins outside the system. But when toxins are flowed out through secondary organs of elimination these areas become inflamed, irritated, weakened. The results can be skin irritations, sinusitis or a whole host of other "itises" depending on the area involved, bacterial or viral infections, asthma. When excess toxemia is deposited instead of eliminated, the results can be arthritis if toxins are stored in joints, rheumatism if in muscle tissues, cysts and benign tumors. And if toxins weaken the body's immune response, cancer.

The liver and the kidneys, the two heroic organs of detoxification, are the most important ones; these jointly act as filters to purify the blood. Hygienists pay a lot of attention to these organs, the liver especially.

In an ideal world, the liver and kidneys would keep up with their job for 80 years or more before even beginning to tire. In this ideal world, the food would of course, be very nutritious and free of pesticide residues, the air and water would be pure, people would not denature their food and turn it into junk. In this perfect world everyone would get moderate exercise into old age, and live virtually without stress. In this utopian vision, the average healthy productive life span would approach a century, entirely without using food supplements or vitamins. In this world doctors would have next to no work other than repairing traumatic injuries, because everyone would be healthy. But this is not the way it is.

In our less-than-ideal world virtually everything we eat is denatured, processed, fried, salted, sweetened, preserved; thus more stress is placed on the liver and kidneys than nature designed them to handle. Except for a few highly fortunate individuals blessed with an incredible genetic endowment that permits them to live to age 99 on moose meat, well-larded white flour biscuits, coffee with evaporated milk and sugar, brandy and cigarettes (we've all heard of someone like this), most peoples' liver and kidneys begin to break down prematurely. Thus doctoring has become a financially rewarding profession.

Most people overburden their organs of elimination by eating whatever they feel like eating whenever they feel like it. Or, they irresponsibly eat whatever is served to them by a mother, wife, institution or cook because doing so is easy or expected. Eating is a very habitual and unconscious activity; frequently we continue to eat as adults whatever our mother fed us as a child. I consider it unsurprising that when people develop the very same disease conditions as their parents. they wrongly assume the cause is genetic inheritance, when actually it was just because they were putting their feet under the same table as their parents.

Toxemia also comes about from following the wrongheaded recommendations of allopathic-inspired nutritional texts and licensed dietitians. For example, people believe they should eat one food from each of the four so-called basic food groups at each meal, thinking they are doing the right thing for their health by having four colors of food on every plate, when they really aren't. What they have actually done is force their bodies to attempt the digestion of indigestible food combinations, and the resulting indigestion creates massive doses of toxins. I'll have a lot more to say about that later when I discuss the art of food combining.

Table 1: The Actual Food Groups

Starches	Proteins	Fats	Sugars	Watery Vegetables
bread	meats	butter	honey	zucchini
potatoes	eggs	oils	fruit	green beans
noodles	fish	lard	sugar	tomatoes
manioc/yuca	most nuts	nuts	molasses	peppers
baked goods	dry beans	avocado	malt syrup	eggplant
grains	nut butters		maple syrup	radish
winter squash	split peas		dried fruit	rutabaga
parsnips	lentils		melons	turnips
sweet potatoes	soybeans		carrot juice	Brussels sprouts
yams	tofu		beet juice	celery
taro root	tempeh			cauliflower
plantains	wheat grass juice			broccoli
beets	"green" drinks			okra
	spirulina			lettuce
	algae			endive
	yeast			cabbage
	dairy			carrots

Standard dietitians divide our foods into four basic food groups and recommend the ridiculous practice of mixing them at every meal. This guarantees indigestion and lots of business for the medical profession. This chart[*] illustrates the actual food groups. It is usually a poor practice to mix different foods from one group with those from another.   [*] Page 33

The Digestive Process

After we have eaten our four-color meal—often we do this in a hurry, without much chewing, under a lot of stress, or in the presence of negative emotions—we give no thought to what becomes of our food once it has been swallowed. We have been led to assume that anything put in the mouth automatically gets digested flawlessly, is efficiently absorbed into the body where it nourishes our cells, with the waste products being eliminated completely by the large intestine. This vision of efficiency may exist in the best cases but for most there is many a slip between the table and the toilet. Most bodies are not optimally efficient at performing all the required functions, especially after years of poor living habits, stress, fatigue, and aging. To the Natural Hygienist, most disease begins and ends with our food; most of our healing efforts are focused on improving the process of digestion.

Digestion means chemically changing the foods we eat into substances that can pass into the blood stream and circulate through the body where nutrition is used for bodily functions. Our bodies use nutritional substances for fuel, for repair and rebuilding, and to conduct an incredibly complex biochemistry. Scientists are still busily engaged in trying to understand the chemical mysteries of our bodies. But as bewildering as the chemistry of life is, the chemistry of digestion itself is actually a relatively simple process, and doctors have had a fairly good understanding of for many decades.

Though relatively straightforward, a lot can and does go wrong with digestion. The body breaks down foods with a series of different enzymes that are mixed with food at various points as it passes from mouth to stomach to small intestine. An enzyme is a large, complex molecule that has the ability to chemically change other large, complex molecules without being changed itself. Digestive enzymes perform relatively simple functions—breaking large molecules into smaller parts that can dissolve in water.

Digestion starts in the mouth when food is mixed with ptyalin, an enzyme secreted by the salivary glands. Pylatin converts insoluble starches into simple sugars. If the digestion of starchy foods is impaired, the body is less able to extract the energy contained in our foods, while far worse from the point of view of the genesis of diseases, undigested starches pass through the stomach and into the gut where they ferment and thereby create an additional toxic burden for the liver to process. And fermenting starches also create gas.

As we chew our food it gets mixed with saliva; as we continue to chew the starches in the food are converted into sugar. There is a very simple experiment you can conduct to prove to yourself how this works. Get a plain piece of bread, no jam, no butter, plain, and without swallowing it or allowing much of it to pass down the throat, begin to chew it until it seems to literally dissolve. Pylatin works fast in our mouths so you may be surprised at how sweet the taste gets. As important as chewing is, I have only run into about one client in a hundred that actually makes an effort to consciously chew their food.

Horace Fletcher, whose name has become synonymous with the importance of chewing food well (Fletcherizing), ran an experiment on a military population in Canada. He required half his experimental group to chew thoroughly, and the other half to gulp things down as usual. His study reports significant improvement in the overall health and performance of the group that persistently chewed. Fletcher's report recommended that every mouthful be chewed 50 times for half a minute before being swallowed. Try it, you might be very surprised at what a beneficial effect such a simple change in your approach to eating can make. Not only will you have less intestinal gas, if overweight you will probably find yourself getting smaller because your blood sugar will elevate quicker as you are eating and thus your sense of hunger will go away sooner. If you are very thin and have difficulty gaining weight you may find that the pounds go on easier because chewing well makes your body more capable of actually assimilating the calories you are consuming.

A logical conclusion from this data is that anything that would prevent or reduce chewing would be unhealthful. For example, food eaten when too hot tends to be gulped down. The same tends to happen when food is seasoned with fresh Jalapeno or habaneo peppers. People with poor teeth should blend or mash starchy foods and then gum them thoroughly to mix them with saliva. Keep in mind that even so-called protein foods such as beans often contain large quantities of starches and the starch portion of protein foods is also digested in the mouth.

Once the food is in the stomach, it is mixed with hydrochloric acid, secreted by the stomach itself, and pepsin, an enzyme. Together these break proteins down into water-soluble amino acids. To accomplish this the stomach muscles agitate the food continuously, somewhat like a washing machine. This extended churning forms a kind of ball in the stomach called a bolis.

Many things can and frequently do go wrong at this stage of the digestive process. First, the stomach's very acid environment inactivates pylatin, so any starch not converted to sugar in the mouth does not get properly processed thereafter. And the most dangerous misdigestion comes from the sad fact that cooked proteins are relatively indigestible no matter how strong the constitution, no matter how concentrated the stomach acid or how many enzymes present. It is quite understandable to me that people do not wish to accept this fact. After all, cooked proteins are so delicious, especially cooked red meats and the harder, more flavorful fishes.

To appreciate this, consider how those enzymes that digest proteins work. A protein molecule is a large, complex string of amino acids, each linked to the next in a specific order. Suppose there are only six amino acids: 1, 2, 3, 4, 5, and 6. So a particular (imaginary) protein could be structured: 1, 4, 4, 6, 2, 3, 5, 4, 2, 3, 6, 1, 1, 2, 3, etc. Thus you should see that by combining a limited number of amino acids there can be a virtually infinite number of proteins.

But proteins are rarely water soluble. As I said a few paragraphs back, digestion consists of rendering insoluble foods into water-soluble substances so they can pass into the blood stream and be used by the body's chemistry. To make them soluble, enzymes break down the proteins, separating the individual amino acids one from the other, because amino acids are soluble. Enzymes that digest proteins work as though they are mirror images of a particular amino acid. They fit against a particular amino acid like a key fits into a lock. Then they break the bonds holding that amino acid to others in the protein chain, and then, what I find so miraculous about this process, the enzyme is capable of finding yet another amino acid to free, and then yet another.

So with sufficient churning in an acid environment, with enough time (a few hours), and enough enzymes, all the recently eaten proteins are decomposed into amino acids and these amino acids pass into the blood where the body recombines them into structures it wants to make. And we have health. But when protein chains are heated, the protein structures are altered into physical shapes that the enzymes can't "latch" on to. The perfect example of this is when an egg is fried. The egg white is albumen, a kind of protein. When it is heated, it shrivels up and gets hard. While raw and liquid, it is easily digestible. When cooked, largely indigestible.

Stress also inhibits the churning action in the stomach so that otherwise digestible foods may not be mixed efficiently with digestive enzymes. For all these reasons, undigested proteins may pass into the gut.

Along with undigested starches. When starches convert best to sugars under the alkaline conditions found in the mouth. Once they pass into the acid stomach starch digestion is not as efficient. If starches reach the small intestine they are fermented by yeasts. The products of starch fermentation are only mildly toxic. The gases produced by yeast fermentations usually don't smell particularly bad; bodies that regularly contain starch fermentation usually don't smell particularly bad either. In otherwise healthy people it can take many years of exposure to starch fermentation toxins to produce a life-threatening disease.

But undigested proteins aren't fermented by yeasts, they putrefy in the gut (are attacked by anaerobic bacteria). Many of the waste products of anaerobic putrefaction are highly toxic and evil smelling; when these toxins are absorbed through the small or large intestines they are very irritating to the mucous membranes, frequently contributing to or causing cancer of the colon. Protein putrefaction may even cause psychotic symptoms in some individuals. Meat eaters often have a very unpleasant body odor even when they are not releasing intestinal gasses.

Adding a heavy toxic burden from misdigested foods to the normal toxic load a body already has to handle creates a myriad of unpleasant symptoms, and greatly shortens life. But misdigestion also carries with it a double whammy; fermenting and/or putrefying foods immediately interfere with the functioning of another vital organ–the large intestine–and cause constipation.

Most people don't know what the word constipation really means. Not being able to move one's bowels is only the most elementary type of constipation. A more accurate definition of constipation is "the retention of waste products in the large intestine beyond the time that is conducive to health." Properly digested food is not sticky and exits the large intestine quickly. But improperly digested food (or indigestible food) gradually coats the large intestine, making an ever-thicker lining that interferes with the intestine's functioning. Far worse, this coating steadily putrefies, creating additional highly-potent toxins. Lining the colon with undigested food can be compared to the mineral deposits filling in the inside of an old water pipe, gradually choking off the flow. In the colon, this deposit can become rock-hard, just like water pipe scale.

Since the large intestine is also an organ that removes moisture and water-soluble minerals from the food and moves them into the blood stream, when the large intestine is lined with putrefying undigested food waste, the toxins of this putrefaction are also steadily moved into the bloodstream and place an even greater burden on the liver and kidneys, accelerating their breakdown, accelerating the aging process and contributing to a lot of interesting and unpleasant symptoms that keep doctors busy and financially solvent. I'll have quite a bit more to say about colon cleansing later.

The Progress *of* Disease: Irritation, Enervation, Toxemia

Disease routinely lies at the end of a three-part chain that goes: irritation or sub-clinical malnutrition, enervation, toxemia. Irritations are something the person does to themselves or something that happens around them. Stresses, in other words.

Mental stressors include strong negative emotional states such as anger, fear, resentment, hopelessness, etc. Behind most diseases it is common to find a problematic mind churning in profound confusion, one generated by a character that avoids responsibility. There may also be job stress or ongoing hostile relationships, often within the family.

Indigestible foods and misdigestion are also stressful irritations, as are mild recreational poisons such as "soft" drugs, tobacco and alcohol. Opiates are somewhat more toxifying, primarily because they paralyze the gut and induce profound constipation. Stimulants like cocaine and amphetamines are the most damaging recreational drugs; these are highly toxic and rapidly shorten life.

Repeated irritations and/or malnutrition eventually produce enervation. The old-time hygienists defined enervation as a lack of or decline in an unmeasurable phenomena, "nerve energy." They viewed the functioning of vital organs as being controlled by or driven by nerve force, sometimes called life force or élan vital. Whatever this vital force actually is, it can be observed and subjectively measured by comparing one person with another. Some people are full of it and literally sparkle with overflowing energy. Beings like this make everyone around them feel good because they somehow momentarily give energy to those endowed with less. Others possess very little and dully plod through life.

As vital force drops, the overall efficiency of all the body's organs correspondingly decline. The pancreas creates less digestive enzymes; the thymus secretes less of its vital hormones that mobilize the immune system; the pituitary makes less growth hormone so the overall repair and rebuilding of cells and tissues slows correspondingly; and so forth. It does not really matter if there is or is not something called nerve energy that can or cannot be measured in a laboratory. Vital force is observable to many people. However, it is measurable by laboratory test that after repeated irritation the overall functioning of the essential organs and glands does deteriorate.

Enervation may develop so gradually that it progresses below the level of awareness of the person, or times of increased enervation can be experienced as a complaint—as a lack of energy, as tiredness, as difficulties digesting, as a new inability to handle a previously-tolerated insult like alcohol.

Long-term consumption of poor-quality food causes enervation. The body is a carbon/oxygen engine designed to run efficiently only on highly nutritious food and this aspect of human genetic programming cannot be changed significantly by adaptation. Given enough generations a human gene pool can adapt to extracting its nutrition from a different group of foods. For example, a group of isolated Fijians currently enjoying long healthy lives eating a diet of seafoods and tropical root crops could suddenly be moved to the highlands of Switzerland and forced to eat the local fare or starve. But most of the Fijians would not have systems adept at making those enzymes necessary to digest cow's milk. So the transplanted Fijians would experience many generations of poorer health and shorter life spans until their genes had been selected for adaptation to the new dietary. Ultimately their descendants could become uniformly healthy on rye bread and dairy products just like the highland Swiss were.

However, modern industrial farming and processing of foodstuffs significantly contributes to mass, widespread enervation in two ways. Humans will probably adjust to the first; the second will, I'm sure, prove insurmountable. First, industrially processed foods are a recent invention and our bodies have not yet adapted to digesting them. In a few more generations humans might be able to accomplish that and public health could improve on factory food. In the meanwhile, the health of humans has declined. Industrially farmed foods have also been lowered in nutritional content compared to what food could be. I gravely doubt if any biological organism can ever adapt to an overall dietary that contains significantly lowered levels of nutrition. I will explain this more fully in the chapter on diet.

Secondary Eliminations Are Disease

However the exact form the chain from irritation or malnutrition to enervation progresses, the ultimate result is an increased level of toxemia, placing an eliminatory burden on the liver and kidneys in excess of their ability. Eventually these organs begin to weaken. Decline of liver and/or kidney function threatens the stability and purity of blood chemistry. Rather than risk complete incapacitation or death from self-poisoning, the overloaded, toxic body, guided by its genetic predisposition and the nature of the toxins (what was eaten, in what state of stress), cleverly channels surplus toxins into its first line of defense–alternative or secondary elimination systems.

Most non-life-threatening yet highly annoying disease conditions originate as secondary eliminations. For example, the skin was designed to sweat, elimination of fluids. Toxemia is often pushed out the sweat glands and is recognized as an unpleasant body odor. A healthy, non-toxic body smells sweet and pleasant (like a newborn baby's body) even after exercise when it has been sweating heavily. Other skin-like organs such as the sinus tissues, were designed to secrete small amounts of mucus for lubrication. The lungs eliminate used air and the tissues are lubricated with mucus-like secretions too. These secretions are types of eliminations, but are not intended for the elimination of toxins. When toxins are discharged in mucus through tissues not designed to handle them, the tissues themselves become irritated, inflamed, weakened and thus much more subject to bacterial or viral infection. Despite this danger, not eliminating surplus toxins carries with it the greater penalty of serious disability or death. Because of this liability, the body, in its wisdom, initially chooses secondary elimination routes as far from vital tissues and organs as possible. Almost inevitably the skin or skin-like mucus membranes such as the sinuses, or lung tissues become the first line of defense.

Thus the average person's disease history begins with colds, flu, sinusitis, bronchitis, chronic cough, asthma, rashes, acne, eczema, psoriasis. If these secondary eliminations are suppressed with drugs (either from the medical doctor or with over the counter remedies), if the eating or lifestyle habits that created the toxemia are not changed, or if the toxic load increases beyond the limits of this technique, the body then begins to store toxins in fat or muscle tissues or the joint cavities, overburdens the kidneys, creates cysts, fibroids, and benign tumors to store those toxins. If toxic overload continues over a longer time the body will eventually have to permit damages to vital tissues, and life-threatening conditions develop.

Hygienic doctors always stress that disease is remedial effort. Illness comes from the body's best attempt to lighten its toxic load without immediately threatening its survival. The body always does the very best it can to remedy toxemia given its circumstances, and it should be commended for these efforts regardless of how uncomfortable they might be to the person inhabiting the body. Symptoms of secondary elimination are actually a positive thing because they are the body's efforts to lessen a dangerously toxic condition. Secondary eliminations shouldn't be treated immediately with a drug to suppress the process. If you squelch the bodies best and least-life-threatening method to eliminate toxins, the body will ultimately have to resort to another more dangerous though probably less immediately uncomfortable channel.

The conventional medical model does not view disease this way and sees the symptoms of secondary elimination as the disease itself. So the conventional doctor takes steps to halt the body's remedial efforts, thus stopping the undesirable symptom and then, the symptom gone, proclaims the patient cured. Actually, the disease is the cure.

A common pattern of symptom suppression under the contemporary medical model is this progression: treat colds with antihistamines until the body gets influenza; suppress a flu repeatedly with antibiotics and eventually you get pneumonia. Or, suppress eczema with cortisone ointment repeatedly, and eventually you develop kidney disease. Or, suppress asthma with bronkiodialators and eventually you need cortisone to suppress it. Continue treating asthma with steroids and you destroy the adrenals; now the body has become allergic to virtually everything.

The presence of toxins in an organ of secondary elimination is frequently the cause of infection. Sinuses and lungs, inflamed by secondary eliminations, are attacked by viruses or bacteria; infectious diseases of the skin result from pushing toxins out of the skin. More generalized infections also result from toxemia; in this case the immune system has become compromised and the body is overwhelmed by an organism that it normally should be able to resist easily. The wise cure of infections is not to use antibiotics to suppress the bacteria while simultaneously whipping the immune system; most people, including most medical doctors, do not realize that antibiotics also goose the immune system into super efforts. But when one chooses to whip a tired horse, eventually the exhausted animal collapses and cannot rise again no matter how vigorously it is beaten. The wise cure is to detoxify the body, a step that simultaneously eliminates secondary eliminations and rebuilds the immune system.

The wise way to deal with the body's eliminative efforts is to accept that disease is an opportunity to pay the piper for past indiscretions. You should go to bed, rest, and drink nothing but water or dilute juice until the condition has passed. This allows the body to conserve its vital energy, direct this energy toward healing the disordered body part, and catch up on its waste disposal. In this way you can help your body, be in harmony with its efforts instead of working against it which is what most people do.

Please forgive another semi-political polemic here, but in my practice I have often been amazed to hear my clients complain that they have not the time nor the ability to be patient with their body, to rest it through an illness because they have a job they can't afford to miss or responsibilities they can't put down. This is a sad commentary on the supposed wealth and prosperity of the United States. In our country most people are enslaved by their debts, incurred because they had been enthralled by the illusion of happiness secured by the possession of material things. Debt slaves believe they cannot miss a week of work. People who feel they can't afford to be sick think they can afford to live on pills. So people push through their symptoms by sheer grit for years on end, and keep that up until their exhausted horse of a body breaks down totally and they find themselves in the hospital running up bills to the tune of several thousand dollars a day. But these very same people do not think they can afford the loss of a few hundred dollars of current income undertaking some virtually harmless preventative maintenance on their bodies.

Given half a chance the body will throw off toxic overburdens and cleanse itself. And once the body has been cleansed of toxemia, disagreeable symptoms usually cease. This means that to make relatively mild but unwanted symptoms lessen and ultimately stop it is merely necessary to temporarily cut back food intake, eating only what does not cause toxemia. These foods I classify as cleansing, such as raw fruits and vegetables and their juices. If the symptoms are extreme, are perceived as overwhelming or are actually life-threatening, detoxification can be speeded up by dropping back to only dilute raw juices or vegetable broth made only from greens, without eating the solids. In the most extreme cases hygienists use their most powerful medicine: a long fast on herb teas, or just water. I will have a lot to say about fasting, later.

When acutely ill, the most important thing to do is to just get out of the body's way, and let it heal itself. In our ignorance we are usually our own worst enemy in this regard. We have been very successfully conditioned to think that all symptoms are bad. But I know from experience that people can and do learn a new way of viewing the body, an understanding that puts them at cause over their own body. It allows you to be empowered in one more area of life instead of being dependent and at the mercy of other peoples decisions about your body.

Finally, and this is why natural medicine is doubly unpopular, to prevent the recurrence of toxemia and acute disease states, person must discover what they are doing wrong and change their life. Often as not this means elimination of the person's favorite (indigestible) foods and/or (stress-producing) bad habits. Naturally, I will have a lot more to say about this later, too.

Chapter Three

Fasting

From The Hygienic Dictionary

Cure. [1] There is no "cure" for disease; fasting is not a cure. Fasting facilitates natural healing processes. Foods do not cure. Until we have discarded our faith in cures, there can be no intelligent approach to the problems presented by suffering and no proper use of foods by those who are ill. *Herbert Shelton, The Hygienic System, v. 3, Fasting and Sunbathing.* [2] All cure starts from within out and from the head down and in reverse order as the symptoms have appeared. *Hering's Law of Cure.* [3] Life is made up of crises. The individual establishes a standard of health peculiarly his own, which must vary from all other standards as greatly as his personality varies from others. The individual standard may be such as to favor the development of indigestion, catarrh, gout, rheumatic and glandular inflammations, tubercular developments, congestions, sluggish secretions and excretions, or inhibitions of various functions, both mental and physical, wherever the environmental or habit strain is greater than usual. The standard of resistance may be opposed so strenuously by habits and unusual physical agencies–that the body breaks down under the strain. This is a crisis. Appetite fails, discomfort or pain forces rest, and, as a result of physiological rest (fasting) and physical rest (rest from daily work and habits), a readjustment takes place, and the patient is "cured." This is what the profession and the people call a cure, and it is for the time being–until an unusual enervation is brought on from accident or dissipation; then another crisis. These crises are the ordinary sickness of all communities– all catalogued diseases. When the cold is gone or the hay-fever fully relieved, it does not mean the patient is cured. Indeed, he is as much diseased as before he suffered the attack–the crisis–and he never will be cured until the habits of life that keep up toxin poisoning are corrected. To recover from a crisis is not a cure; the tendency is back to the individual standard; hence all crises are self-limited, unless nature by maltreatment is prevented from reacting. All so-called healing systems ride to glory on the backs of self-limited crises, and the self-deluded doctors and their credulous clients, believe, when the crises are past, that a cure has been wrought, whereas the real truth is that the treatment may have delayed reaction. This is largely true of anything that has been done except rest. A cure consists in changing the manner of living to such a rational standard that full resistance and a balanced metabolism is established. I suppose it is not quite human to expect those of a standardized school of healing to give utterance to discovered truth which, if accepted by the people, would rob them of the glory of being curers of disease. Indeed, nature, and nature only, cures; and as for crises, they come and go, whether or not there is a doctor or healer within a thousand miles.

Dr. John. H. Tilden, Impaired Health: Its Cause and Cure, 1921.

The accelerated healing process that occurs during fasting can scarcely be believed by a person who has not fasted. No matter how gifted the writer, the experiential reality of fasting cannot be communicated. The great novelist Upton Sinclair wrote a book about fasting and it failed to convince the multitudes. But once a person has fasted long enough to be certain of what their own body can do to fix itself, they acquire a degree of independence little known today. Many of those experienced with fasting no longer dread being without health insurance and feel far less need for a doctor or of having a regular checkup. They know with certainty that if something degenerates in their body, their own body can fix it by itself.

Like Upton Sinclair and many others who largely failed before me, I am going to try to convince you of the virtues of fasting by urging you to try fasting yourself. If you will but try you will be changed for the better for the rest of your life. If you do not try, you will never know.

To prompt your first step on this health-freedom road, I ask you to please carefully consider the importance of this fact: the body's routine energy budget includes a very large allocation for the daily digestion and assimilation of the food you eat. You may find my estimate surprising, but about one-third of a fairly sedentary person's entire energy consumption goes into food processing. Other uses for the body's energy include the creation or rebuilding of tissues, detoxification, moving (walking, running, etc.), talking, producing hormones, etc. Digestion is one aspect of the body's efforts that we can readily control, it is the key to having or losing health.

The Effort *of* Digestion

Digestion is a huge, unappreciated task, unappreciated because few of us are aware of its happening in the same way we are aware of making efforts to use our voluntary muscles when working or exercising. Digestion begins in the mouth with thorough chewing. If you don't think chewing is effort, try making coleslaw in your own mouth. Chew up at least half a big head of cabbage and three big carrots that have not been shredded. Grind each bit until it liquefies and has been thoroughly mixed with saliva. I guarantee that if you even finish the chore your jaw will be tired and you will have lost all desire to eat anything else, especially if it requires chewing.

Making the saliva you just used while chewing the cabbage is by itself, a huge and unappreciated chemical effort.

Once in the stomach, chewed food has to be churned in order to mix it with hydrochloric acid, pepsin, and other digestive enzymes. Manufacturing these enzymes is also considerable work! Churning is even harder work than chewing but normally, people are unaware of its happening. While the stomach is churning (like a washing machine) a large portion of the blood supply is redirected from the muscles in the extremities to the stomach and intestines to aid in this process. Anyone who has tried to go for a run, or take part in any other strenuous physical activity immediately after a large meal feels like a slug and wonders why they just can't make their legs move the way they usually do. So, to assist the body while it is digesting, it is wise to take a siesta as los Latinos do instead of expecting the blood to be two places at once like *los norteamericanos.*

After the stomach is through churning, the partially digested food is moved into the small intestine where it is mixed with more pancreatin secreted by the pancreas, and with bile from the gall bladder. Pancreatin further solubilizes proteins. Bile aids in the digestion of fatty foods. Manufacturing bile and pancreatic enzymes is also a lot of effort. Only after the carbohydrates (starches and sugars), proteins and fats have been broken down into simpler water soluble food units such as simple sugars, amino acids and fatty acids, can the body pass these nutrients into the blood thorough the little projections in the small intestines called villi.

The leftovers, elements of the food that can't be solubilized plus some remaining liquids, are passed into the large intestine. There, water and the vital mineral salts dissolved in that water, are extracted and absorbed into the blood stream through thin permeable membranes. Mucous is also secreted in the large intestine to facilitate passage of the dryish remains. This is an effort. (Intestinal mucous can become a route of secondary elimination, especially during fasting. While fasting, it is essential to take steps to expel toxic mucous in the colon before the poisons are re adsorbed.) The final residue, now called fecal matter, is squeezed along the length of the large intestines and passes out the rectum.

If all the digestive processes have been efficient there now are an abundance of soluble nutrients for the blood stream to distribute to hungry cells throughout the body. It is important to understand the process at least on the level of oversimplification just presented in order to begin to understand better how health is lost or regained through eating, digestion, and elimination. And most importantly, through not eating.

How Fasting Heals

It's an old hygienic maxim that the doctor does not heal, the medicines do not heal, only the body heals itself. If the body can't heal then nothing can heal it. The body always knows best what it needs and what to do.

But healing means repairing damaged organs and tissues and this takes energy, while a sick body is already enervated, weakened and not coping with its current stressors. If the sick person could but somehow increase the body's energy resources sufficiently, then a slowly healing body could heal faster while a worsening one, or one that was failing or one that was not getting better might heal.

Fasting does just that. To whatever degree food intake is reduced the body's digestive workload is proportionately reduced and it will naturally, and far more intelligently than any physician could order, redirect energy to wherever it decides that energy is most needed. A fasting body begins accessing nutritional reserves (vitamins and minerals) previously stored in the tissues and starts converting body fat into sugar for energy fuel. During a time of water fasting, sustaining the body's entire energy and nutritional needs from reserves and fat does require a small effort, but far less effort than eating. I would guess a fasting body used about five percent of its normal daily energy budget on nutritional concerns rather than the 33 percent it needs to process new food. Thus, water fasting puts something like 28 percent more energy at the body's disposal. This is true even though the water faster may feel weak, energyless.

I would worry if sick or toxic fasters did not complain about their weakness. They should expect to feel energyless. In fact, the more internal healing and detoxification the body requires, the tireder the faster feels because the body is very hard at work internally. A great deal of the body's energy will go toward boosting the immune system if the problem is an infection. Liberated energy can also be used for healing damaged parts, rebuilding failing organs, for breaking down and eliminating deposits of toxic materials. Only after most of the healing has occurred does a faster begin to feel energetic again. Don't expect to feel anything but tired and weak.

The only exception to this would be a person who has already significantly detoxified and healed their body by previous fasting, or the rare soul that has gone from birth through adulthood enjoying extraordinarily good nutrition and without experiencing the stressors of improper digestion. When one experienced faster I know finds himself getting "run down" or catching a cold, he quits eating until he feels really well. Instead of feeling weak as most fasters do, as each of the first four or five days of water fasting pass, he experiences a resurgence of more and more energy. On the first fasting day he would usually feel rotten, which was why he started fasting in the first place. On the second fasting day he'd feel more alert and catch up on his paper work. By his third day on only water he would be out doing hard physical chores like cutting the grass, splitting wood or weeding his vegetable garden. Day four would also be an energetic one, but if the fast extended beyond that, lowering blood sugar would begin to make him tired and he'd feel forced to begin laying down.

After a day of water fasting the average person's blood sugar level naturally drops; making a faster feel somewhat tired and "spacey," so a typical faster usually begins to spend much more time resting, further reducing the amount of energy being expended on moving the body around, serendipitously redirecting even more of the body's energy budget toward healing. By the end of five or six days on water, I estimate that from 40 to 50 percent of the body's available energy is being used for healing, repair and detoxification.

The amount of work that a fasting body's own healing energy can do and what it feels like to be there when it is happening is incredible. But you can't know it if you haven't felt it. So hardly anyone in our present culture knows.

As I mentioned in the first chapter, at Great Oaks School I apprenticed myself to the traveling masters of virtually every system of natural healing that existed during the '70s. I observed every one of them at work and tried most of them on my clients. After all that I can say with experience that I am not aware of any other healing tool that can be so effective as the fast.

Essentials of a Successful, Safe Fast

1. Fast in a bright airy room, with exceptionally good ventilation, because fasters not only need a lot of fresh air; their bodies give off powerfully offensive odors.

2. Sun bathe if possible in warm climates for 10 to 20 minutes in the morning before the sun gets too strong.

3. Scrub/massage the skin with a dry brush, stroking toward the heart, followed by a warm water shower two to four times a day to assist the skin in eliminating toxins. If you are too weak to do this, have an assisted bed bath.

4. Have two enemas daily for the first week of a fast and then once daily until the fast is terminated.

5. Insure a harmonious environment with supportive people or else fast alone if you are experienced. Avoid well-meaning interference or anxious criticism at all cost. The faster becomes hypersensitive to others' emotions.

6. Rest profoundly except for a short walk of about 200 yards morning and night.

7. Drink water! At least three quarts every day. Do not allow yourself to become dehydrated!

8. Control yourself! Break a long fast on diluted non-sweet fruit juice such as grapefruit juice, sipped a teaspoon at a time, no more than eight ounces at a time no oftener than every 2 or 3 hours. The second day you eat, add small quantities of fresh juicy fruit to the same amount of juice you took the day before no oftener than every 3 hours. By small quantities I mean half an apple or the equivalent. On the third day of eating, add small quantities of vegetable juice and juicy vegetables such as tomatoes and cucumbers.

Control yourself! The second week after eating resumed add complex vegetable salads plus more complex fruit salads. Do not mix fruit and vegetables at meals. The third week add raw nuts and seeds no more than 1/2 ounce three times daily. Add 1/4 avocado daily. Fourth week increase to 3 ounces of raw soaked nuts and seeds daily and 1/2 avocado daily. Cooked grains may also be added, along with steamed vegetables and vegetable soups.

The Prime Rules *of* Fasting

Another truism of natural hygiene is that we dig our own graves with our teeth. It is sad but true that almost all eat too much quantity of too little quality. Dietary excesses are the main cause of death in North America. Fasting balances these excesses. If people were to eat a perfect diet and not overeat, fasting would rarely be necessary.

There are two essential rules of fasting. If these rules are ignored or broken, fasting itself can be life threatening. But if the rules are followed, fasting presents far less risk than any other important medical procedure with a far greater likelihood of a positive outcome. And let me stress here, there is no medical procedure without risk. Life itself is fraught with risk, it is a one-way ticket from birth to death, with no certainty as to when the end of the line will be reached. But in my opinion, when handling degenerative illness and infections, natural hygiene and fasting usually offer the best hope of healing with the least possible risk.

The first vital concern is the duration of the fast. Two eliminatory processes go on simultaneously while fasting. One is the dissolving and elimination of the excess, toxic or dysfunctional deposits in the body, and second process, the gradual exhaustion of the body's stored nutritional reserves. The fasting body first consumes those parts of the body that are unhealthy; eventually these are all gone. Simultaneously the body uses up stored fat and other reserve nutritional elements. A well-fed reasonably healthy body usually has enough stored nutrition to fast for quite a bit longer than it takes to "clean house."

While house cleaning is going on the body uses its reserves to rebuild organs and rejuvenate itself. Rebuilding starts out very slowly but the repairs increase at an ever-accelerating rate. The "overhaul" can last only until the body has no more reserves. Because several weeks of fasting must pass by before the "overhaul" gets going full speed, it is wise to continue fasting as long as possible so as to benefit from as much rejuvenation as possible.

It is best not to end the fast before all toxic or dysfunctional deposits are eliminated, or before the infection is overcome, or before the cause for complaint has been healed. The fast must be ended when most of the body's essential-to-life stored nutritional reserves are exhausted. If the fast goes beyond this point, starvation begins.

Then, fasting-induced organic damage can occur, and death can follow, usually several weeks later. Almost anyone not immediately close to death has enough stored nutrition to water fast for ten days to two weeks. Most reasonably healthy people have sufficient reserves to water fast for a month. Later I will explain how a faster can somewhat resupply their nutritional reserves while continuing to fast, and thus safely extend the fasting period.

The second essential concern has to do with adjusting the intensity of the fast. Some individuals are so toxic that the waste products released during a fast are too strong, too concentrated or too poisonous for the organs of elimination to handle safely, or to be handled within the willingness of the faster to tolerate the discomforts that toxic releases generate. The highly-toxic faster may even experience life-threatening symptoms such as violent asthma attacks. This kind of faster has almost certainly been dangerously ill before the fast began. Others, though not dangerously sick prior to fasting, may be nearly as toxic and though not in danger of death, they may not be willing to tolerate the degree of discomfort fasting can trigger. For this reason I recommend that if at all possible, before undertaking a fast the person eat mostly raw foods for two months and clean up all addictions. This will give the body a chance to detoxify significantly before the water fast is started, and will make water fasting much more comfortable. Seriously, dangerously ill people should only fast with experienced guidance, so the rapidity of their detoxification process may be adjusted to a lower level if necessary.

A fast of only one week can accomplish a significant amount of healing. Slight healing does occur on shorter fasts, but it is much more difficult to see or feel the results. Many people experience rapid relief from acute headache pain or digestive distress such as gas attacks, mild gallbladder pain, stomach aches, etc., after only one day's abstention from food. In one week of fasting a person can relieve more dangerous conditions such as arthritic pain, rheumatism, kidney pain, and many symptoms associated with allergic reactions. But even more fasting time is generally needed for the body to completely heal serious diseases. That's because eliminating life-threatening problems usually involve rebuilding organs that aren't functioning too well. Major rebuilding begins only after major detoxification has been accomplished, and this takes time.

Yes, even lost organ function can be partially or completely restored by fasting. Aging and age-related degeneration is progressive, diminishing organ functioning. Organs that make digestive enzymes secrete less enzymes. The degenerated immune system loses the ability to mobilize as effectively when the body is attacked. Liver and kidney efficiency declines. The adrenals tire, becoming incapable of dumping massive amounts of stress-handling hormones or of repeating that effort time after time without considerable rest in between. The consequences of these inter-dependent deterioration's is a cascade of deterioration that contributes to even more rapid deterioration's. The name for this cascading process is aging. Its inevitable result–death.

Fasting can, to a degree, reverse aging. Because fasting improves organ functioning, it can slow down aging.

Fasters are often surprised that intensified healing can be uncomfortable. They have been programmed by our culture and by allopathic doctors to think that if they are doing the right thing for their bodies they should feel better immediately. I wish it weren't so, but most people have to pay the piper for their dietary indiscretions and other errors in living. There will be aches and minor pains and uncomfortable sensations. More about that later. A rare faster does feel immediately better, and continues to feel ever better by the day, and even has incredible energy while eating nothing, but the majority of us folks just have to tough it out, keeping in mind that the way out is the way through. It is important to remind yourself at times that even with some discomfort and considering the inconvenience of fasting that you are getting off easy–one month of self-denial pays for those years of indulgence and buys a regenerated body.

Length *of the* Fast

How long should a person fast? In cases where there are serious complaints to remedy but where there are no life threatening disease conditions, a good rule of thumb is to fast on water for one complete day (24 hours) for each year that the person has lived. If you are 30 years old, it will take 30 consecutive days of fasting to restore complete health. However, thirty fasting days, done a few days here and a few there won't equal a month of steady fasting; the body accomplishes enormously more in 7 or 14 days of consecutive fasting, than 7 or 14 days of fasting accumulated sporadically, such as one day a week. This is not to say that regular short fasts are not useful medicine. Periodic day-long fasts have been incorporated into many religious traditions, and for good reason; it gives the body one day a week to rest, to be free of digestive obligations, and to catch up on garbage disposal. I heartily recommend it. But it takes many years of unfailingly regular brief fasting to equal the benefits of one, intensive experience.

Fasting on water much longer than fifteen consecutive days may be dangerous for the very sick, (unless under experienced supervision) or too intense for those who are not motivated by severe illness to withstand the discomfort and boredom. However, it is possible to finish a healing process initiated by one long water fast by repeating the fast later. My husband's healing is a good example of this. His health began to noticeably decline about age 38 and he started fasting. He fasted on water 14 to 18 days at a time, once a year, for five consecutive years before most of his complaints and problems entirely vanished.

The longest fast I ever supervised was a 90 day water fast on an extraordinarily obese woman, who at 5' 2" weighed close to 400 pounds. She was a Mormon; generally members of the LDS Church eat a healthier diet than most Americans, but her's included far too much of what I call "healthfood junkfood," in the form of whole grain cakes and cookies, lots of granola made with lots of honey, oil, and dried fruit, lots of honey heaped atop heavily buttered whole grain bread. (I will explain more about the trap of healthfood junkfood later on.) A whole foods relatively meatless diet is far superior to its refined white flour, white sugar and white grease (lard) counterpart, but it still produced a serious health problem in just 30 years of life. Like many women, she expressed love-for-family in the kitchen by serving too-much too-tasty food. The Mormons have a very strong family orientation and this lady was no exception, but she was insecure and unhappy in her marriage and sought consolation in food, eaten far in excess of what her body needed.

On her 90 day water fast she lost about 150 pounds, but was still grossly overweight when the fast ended. Toward the end it became clear that it was unrealistic to try to shrink this woman any closer to normal body weight because to her, fat represented an invaluable insulation or buffer that she was not prepared to give up. As the weight melted away on the fast and she was able to actually feel the outline of a hip bone her neurosis became more and more apparent, and the ability to feel a part of her skeleton was so upsetting to her that her choice was between life threatening obesity and pervasive anxiety.

Her weight was still excessive but the solace of eating was even more important. This woman needed intensive counseling not more fasting. Unfortunately, at the end she choose to remain obese. Fat was much less frightening to her than confronting her emotions and fears. The positive side was that after the fast she was able to maintain her weight at 225 instead of 375 which was an enormous relief to her exhausted heart.

Another client I fasted for 90 days was a 6' 1" tall, chronic schizophrenic man who weighed in at 400 pounds. He was so big he could barely get through my front door, and mine was an extraordinarily wide in what had been an upper-class mansion. This man, now in his mid twenties, had spent his last seven years in a mental institution before his parents decided to give him one last chance by sending to Great Oaks School. The state mental hospitals at that time provided the mentally ill with cigarettes, coffee, and lots of sugary treats, but none of these substances were part of my treatment program so he had a lot of immediate withdrawal to go through. The quickest and easiest way to get him through it was to put him on a water fast after a few days of preparation on raw food.

This was not an easily managed case! He was wildly psychotic, on heavy doses of chloropromazine, with many bizarre behaviors. Besides talking to himself continuously in gibberish, he collected bugs, moss, sticks, piles or dirt, and switched to smoking oak leaves instead of cigarettes. He was such a fire hazard that I had to move him to a downstairs room with concrete floor. Even in the basement he was a fire hazard with his smoking and piles of sticks and other inflammables next to his bed, but all of this debris was his "precious." I knew that I was in for trouble if I disturbed his precious, but the insects and dirt piles seemed to be expanding exponentially.

One day the dirt exceeded my tolerance level. To make a long story short he caught me in the act of cleaning up his precious. Was he furious! All 350 pounds of him! (By this time he had lost 50 pounds.) He barreled into me, fists flying, and knocked me into the pipes next to the furnace and seemed ready to really teach me what was what. I prefer to avoid fights, but if they are inevitable, I can really get into the spirit of the thing. I'd had lots of childhood practice defending myself because I was an incurable tomboy who loved to wrestle; I could usually pin big boys who considered themselves tough. So I began using my fists and what little martial arts training I had to good use. After I hurt him a bit he realized that I was not going to be easily intimidated, and that in fact he was in danger of getting seriously damaged. So he called a truce before either of us were badly beaten up. He had only a few bruises and welts, nothing serious.

After that he refrained from collecting things inside the building (he continued to collect outside). This compromise was fine with me, and the incident allowed me to maintain the authority I needed to bully him into co-operating with the program: taking his vitamins, and sticking to his fast until he finally reached 200 pounds. After 90 days on water he actually looked quite handsome, he no longer smoked, he was off psychotropic medication, and his behaviors were within an acceptable range as long as your expectations were not too high.

He was well enough to live outside a hospital and also clear-headed enough to know that if he let too many people know how well he really was, he might have to give up his mental disability pension and actually become responsible for himself. No way, Jose! This fellow knew a good thing when he saw it. So he continued to pull bizarre stunts just often enough in front of the right audience to keep his disability checks coming in, while managing to act sane enough to be allowed to live comfortably at home instead of in the hospital. By keeping to my program he could stay off mind-numbing psychotropic medication if he kept up his megavitamins and minerals. This compromise was tolerable from his point of view, because there were no side effects like he experienced from his tranquilizers.

It is very rare for a mentally ill person who has spent more than a few months in a mental hospital to ever usefully return to society because they find "mental illness" too rewarding.

My Own 56 Day Long Fast

Fasters go through a lot of different emotional states, these can get intense and do change quite rapidly. The physical body, too, will manifest transitory conditions. Some can be quite uncomfortable. But, I don't want to leave the reader with the impression that fasting is inevitably painful. So I will now recount my own longest fast in detail.

When I did my own 42 day water fast followed by two weeks on carrot juice diluted 50/50 with water, which really amounted to 56 consecutive days, my predominant sensation for the first three days was a desire to eat that was mostly a mental condition, and a lot of rumbling and growling from my stomach. This is not real hunger, just the sounds the stomach likes to make when it is shrinking. After all, this organ is accustomed to being filled at regular intervals, and then, all of a sudden, it gets nothing, so naturally the stomach wants to know what is going on. Once it realizes it is on temporary vacation, the stomach wisely decides to reduce itself to a size suitable for a retired organ. And it shuts up. This process usually takes three to five days and for most people, no further "hunger pangs" are felt until the fast is over.

Real hunger comes only when the body is actually starving. The intense discomforts many people experience upon missing a meal are frequently interpreted as hunger but they aren't. What is actually happening is that their highly toxic bodies are taking the opportunity presented by having missed a meal or two to begin to cleanse. The toxins being released and processed make assorted unpleasant symptoms such as headaches and inability to think clearly. These symptoms can be instantly eliminated by the intake of a bit of food, bringing the detox to a screeching halt.

Two weeks into the fast I experienced sharp abdominal pains that felt like I imagine appendicitis feels, which compelled me toward the nearest toilet in a state of great urgency where I productively busied myself for about half an hour. As I mentioned earlier, I was experimentally adhering to a rigid type of fast of the sort recommended by Dr. Herbert Shelton, a famous advocate of the Natural Hygiene school. Shelton was such a powerful writer and personality that there still exists a Natural Hygiene Society that keeps his books in print and maintains his library. The words "Natural Hygiene" are almost owned by the society like a trademark and they object when anyone describes themselves as a hygienist and then advocates any practice that Dr. Shelton did not approve of.

Per Dr. Shelton, I was going to fast from the time hunger left until the time it returned and I was not going to use any form of colon cleansing. Shelton strongly opposed bowel cleansing so I did no enemas nor colonics, nor herbs, nor clays, nor psyllium seed designed to clean the bowel, etc. Obviously at day 14 the bowel said, enough is enough of this crap, and initiated a goods house cleaning session. When I saw what was eliminated I was horrified to think that I had left that stuff in there for two weeks. I then started to wonder if the Sheltonites were mistaken about this aspect of fasting. Nonetheless, I persevered on the same regimen because my hunger had not returned, my tongue was still thickly coated with foul-smelling, foul-tasting mucus and I still had some fat on my feet that had not been metabolized.

Shelton said that cleansing is not complete until a skeletal condition is reached–that is, absolutely no fat reserves are left. Up until that time I did not even know that I had fat on my feet, but much to my surprise, as the weeks went on, not only did my breasts disappear except for a couple of land marks well-known to my babies, but my ribs and hip bones became positively dangerous to passersby, and my shoes would not stay on my feet. This was not all that surprising because I went from 135 pounds down to 85 on a 5' 7" frame with substantial bone structure.

Toward the end of the fast my eyes became brighter and clearer blue, my skin took on a good texture, my breath finally became sweet, my tongue cleared up and became pink, my mind was clear, and my spiritual awareness and sensitivity was heightened. In other words, I was no longer a walking hulk of stored-up toxemia. I also felt quite weak and had to rest for ten minutes out every hour in horizontal position. (I should have rested much more.) I also required very little sleep, although it felt good to just lie quietly and rest, being aware of what was going on in various parts of my body.

During the last few weeks on water I became very attentive to my right shoulder. Two separate times in the past, while flying head first over the handlebars of my bicycle I had broken my shoulder with considerable tearing of ligaments and tendons. At night when I was totally still I felt a whole crew of pixies and brownies with picks and shovels at work in the joint doing major repair work. This activity was not entirely comfortable, but I knew it was constructive work, not destructive, so I joined the work crew with my mind's eye and helped the work along.

It seemed my visualizations actually did help. Ever since, I've had the fasters I supervised use creative imagery or write affirmations to help their bodies heal. There are lots of books on this subject. I've found that the techniques work far better on a faster than when a person is eating normally.

After breaking the fast it took me six weeks to regain enough strength that I could run my usual distance in my regular time; it took me six months to regain my full 135 pound weight because I was very careful to break the fast slowly and correctly. Coming off water with two weeks on dilute carrot juice I then added small portions of raw food such as apples, raw vegetables, sprouts, vegetable juices, and finally in the fourth week after I began drinking dilute carrot juice, I added seven daily well-chewed almonds to my rebuilding diet. Much later I increased to 14 almonds, but that was the maximum amount of such highly concentrated fare my body wanted digest at one time for over one year. I found I got a lot more miles to the gallon out of the food that I did eat, and did not crave recreational foods. Overall I was very pleased with my educational fast, it had taught me a great deal.

If I had undertaken such a lengthy fast at a time when I was actually ill, and therefore had felt forced into it, my experience could have been different. A positive mental attitude is an essential part of the healing process so fasting should not be undertaken in a negative, protesting mental state. The mind is so powerful that fear or the resistance fear generates can override the healing capacity of the body. For that reason I always recommend that people who consider themselves to be healthy, who have no serious complaints, but who are interested in water fasting, should limit themselves to ten consecutive days or so, certainly never more than 14. Few healthy people, even those with a deep interest in the process, can find enough personal motivation to overcome the extreme boredom of water fasting for longer than that. Healthy people usually begin protesting severely after about two weeks. If there is any one vital rule of fasting, one never should fast over strong, personal protest. Anytime you're fasting and you really desire to quit, you probably should. Unless, of course, you are critically ill. Then you may have no choice—its fast or die.

Common Fasting Complaints And Discomforts

The most frequently heard complaints of fasters are headaches, dry, cracked lips, dizziness, blurred vision with black spots that float, skin rashes, and weakness in the first few days plus what they think is intense hunger. The dizziness and weakness are really real, and are due to increased levels of toxins circulating in the blood and from unavoidably low blood sugar which is a natural consequence of the cessation of eating. The blood sugar does reestablish a new equilibrium in the second and third week of the fast and then, the dizziness may cease, but still, it is important to expect dizziness at the beginning.

It always takes more time for the blood to reach the head on a fast because everything has slowed down, including the rate of the heart beat, so blood pressure probably has dropped as well. If you stand up very quickly you may faint. I repetitively instruct all of my clients to stand up very slowly, moving from a lying to a sitting position, pausing there for ten or twenty seconds, and then rising slowly from a sitting to a standing position. They are told that at the first sign of dizziness they must immediately put their head between their knees so that the head is lower than the heart, or squat/sit down on the floor, I once had a faster who forgot to obey my frequent warnings. About two weeks into a long fast, she got up rapidly from the toilet and felt dizzy. The obvious thing to do was to sit back down on the toilet or lie down on the bath rug on the floor, but no, she decided that because she was dizzy she should rush back to her bed in the adjoining room. She made it as far as the bathroom door and fainted, out cold, putting a deep grove into the drywall with her pretty nose on the way down. We then had to make an unscheduled visit to a nose specialist, who calmly put a tape-wrapped spoon inside her bent-over nose and pried it back to dead center. This was not much fun for either of us; it is well worthwhile preventing such complications.

Other common complaints during the fast include coldness, due to low blood sugar as well as a consequence of weight loss and slowed circulation due to lessened physical activity. People also dislike inactivity which seems excruciatingly boring, and some are upset by weight loss itself. Coldness is best handled with lots of clothes, bedding, hot water bottles or hot pads, and warm baths. Great Oaks School of Health was in Oregon, where the endlessly rainy winters are chilly and the concrete building never seemed to get really warm. I used to dream of moving my fasters to a tropical climate where I could also get the best, ripest fruits to wean them back on to food.

If the fast goes on for more than a week or ten days, many people complain of back discomfort, usually caused by over-worked kidneys. This passes. Hot baths or hot water bottles provide some relief. Drinking more fluids may also help a bit. Nausea is fairly common too, due to toxic discharges from the gall bladder. Drinking lots of water or herbal tea dilutes toxic bile in the stomach and makes it more tolerable.

Very few fasters sleep well and for some reason they expect to, certainly fasters hope to, because they think that if they sleep all night they will better survive one more deadly dull day in a state of relative unconsciousness. They find out much to their displeasure that very little sleep is required on a fast because the body is at rest already. Many fasters sleep only two to four hours but doze frequently and require a great deal of rest. Being mentally prepared for this change of habit is the best handling. Generalized low-grade aches and pains in the area of the diseased organs or body parts are common and can often be alleviated with hot water bottles, warm but not hot bath water and massage. If this type of discomfort exists, it usually lessens with each passing day until it disappears altogether.

Many fasters complain that their vision is blurred, and that they are unable to concentrate. These are really major inconveniences because then fasters can't read or even pay close attention to video-taped movies, and if they can't divert themselves some fasters think they will go stir crazy. They are so addicted to a hectic schedule of doingness, and/or being entertained that they just can't stand just being with themselves, forced to confront and deal with the sensations of their own body, forced to face their own thoughts, to confront their own emotions, many of which are negative. People who are fasting release a lot of mental/emotional garbage at the same time as they let go of old physical garbage. Usually the psychological stuff contributed greatly to their illness and just like the physical garbage and degenerated organs, it all needs to be processed.

One of the most distressing experiences that happen occasionally is hair loss. Deprived of adequate nutrition, the follicles cannot keep growing hair, and the existing hair dies. However, the follicles themselves do not die and once the fast has ended and sufficient nutrition is forthcoming, hair will regrow as well or better than before.

There are also complaints that occur after the fast has been broken. Post-fast cravings, even after only two weeks of deprivation, are to be expected. These may take the form of desires for sweet, sour, salt, or a specific food dreamed of while fasting, like chocolate fudge sundays or just plain toast. Food cravings must be controlled at all costs because if acted upon, each indulgence chips away the health gains of the previous weeks. A single indulgence can be remedied by a day of restricting the diet to juice or raw food. After the repair, the person feels as good as they did when the fast ended. Repeated indulgences will require another extended bout of fasting to repair. It is far better to learn self-control.

The Healing Crisis & Retracing

Certain unpleasant somatics that occur while fasting (or while on a healing diet) may not be dangerous or "bad." Two types, the healing crisis, and retracing, are almost inevitable. A well-educated faster should welcome these discomforts when they happen. The healing crisis (but not retracing) also occurs on a healing diet.

The healing crisis can seem a big surprise to a faster who has been progressing wonderfully. Suddenly, usually after a few days of noticeably increased well-being, they suddenly experience a set of severe symptoms and feel just awful. This is not a setback, not something to be upset or disappointed about, but a healing crisis, actually a positive sign

Healing crises always occur after a period of marked improvement. As the vital force builds up during the healing process, the body decides it now has obtained enough energy to throw off some accumulated toxins, and forcefully pushes them out through a typical and usually previously used route of secondary elimination, such as the nose, lungs, stomach, intestines, skin, or perhaps produces a flu-like experience with fever chills, sweat, aches and pains, etc. Though unpleasant, this experience is to be encouraged; the body has merely accelerated its elimination process. Do not attempt to suppress any of these symptoms, don't even try to moderate fever, which is the body's effective way to burn out a virus or bacteria infection, unless it is a dangerously high fever (over 102 degree Fahrenheit). Fever can be lowered without drugs by putting the person into a cool/cold bath, or using cold towel wraps and cold water sponge baths. The good news is that healing crises usually do not last long, and when they are past you feel better than you did before the crisis.

Asthmatics seem to have the worst crises. I have had asthmatics bring up a quart of obnoxious mucous from their lungs every night for weeks. They have stayed awake all night for three nights continuously coughing and choking on the material that was being eliminated. After that clearing-out process they were able to breathe much more freely. Likewise I have had people who have had sinusitis have nothing but non-stop pussy discharge from their sinuses for three weeks. Some of this would run down the throat and cause nausea. All I could say to encourage the sufferer was that it needed to come out and to please stand aside and let the body work its magic. These fasters were not grateful until the sinus problem that had plagued them since childhood disappeared.

The interesting thing about healing crises are that the symptoms produced retrace earlier complaints; they are almost never something entirely unknown to the patient. Usually they are old, familiar somatics, often complaints that haven't bothered the faster for many years. The reason the symptom is familiar but is not currently a problem is because as the body degenerates it loses vital force; with less vital force it loses the ability to create such acute detoxification episodes in non-life-threatening secondary elimination routes. The degenerated body makes less violent efforts to cleanse, efforts that aren't as uncomfortable. The negative side of this is that instead of creating acute discomfort in peripheral systems, the toxemia goes to more vital organs where it hastens the formation of life-threatening conditions.

There is a very normal and typical progress for each person's fatal illness. Their ultimate disease starts out in childhood or adolescence as acute inflammations of skin-like organs, viral or bacterial infections of the same. Then, as vital force weakens, secondary eliminations are shifted to more vital organs. Allergies or colds stop happening so frequently; the person becomes rheumatic, arthritic or experience weakness in joints, tendons, ligaments, or to have back pains, or to have digestive upsets. These new symptoms are more constant but usually less acute. Ultimately, vital organs begin to malfunction, and serious diseases develop. But a hygienist sees the beginning of fatal diseases such as cancer in adolescent infections and allergies.

Retracing is generally seen only on water fasts, not on extended cleansing diets. The body begins to repair itself by healing conditions in the reverse order to that which they occurred originally. This means that the body would first direct healing toward the lungs if the most recently serious illness was an attack of pneumonia six months previously. In this case you would expect to quickly and intensely experience a mini-case of pneumonia while the body eliminates residues in the lungs that were not completely discharged at the time. Next the body might take you through a period of depression that you had experienced five years in the past. The faster may be profoundly depressed for a few days and come out of it feeling much better. You could then reexperience sensation-states like those caused by recreational drugs you had playfully experimented with ten years previously along with the "trippiness" if it were a hallucinogen, speediness if it was "speed" or the dopiness if it was heroin. Retracing further, the faster might then experience something similar to a raging attack of tonsillitis which you vaguely remember having when you were five years old, but fortunately this time it passes in three days (or maybe six hours), instead of three weeks. This is retracing.

Please do not be surprised or alarmed if it happens to you on a fast, and immediately throw out the baby with the bath water thinking that you are doing the wrong thing because all those old illnesses are coming back to haunt you. It is the body's magnificent healing effort working on your behalf, and for doing it your body deserves lots of "well done", "good body" thoughts rather than gnashing of teeth and thinking what did I do to deserve this. The body won't tell you what you did to deserve this, but it knows and is trying its darndest to undo it.

The Unrelenting Boredom *of* Fasting

Then there's the unrelenting boredom of fasting. Most people have been media junkies since they were kids; the only way they believe they can survive another day of fasting is by diverting their minds with TV. This is far from ideal because often the emotions of a faster are like an open wound and when they resonate with the emotions portrayed on most TV shows, the faster gets into some very unpleasant states that interfere with healing. And the emotions many movies prompt people to sympathetically generate are powerful ones, often highly negative, and contrary to healing. Especially unhelpful are the adrenaline rushes in action movies. But if TV is the best a faster can do, it is far better that someone fast with television programming filling their minds than to not fast at all. I keep a library of positive VHS tapes for these addicts–comedies, stories of heroic over-comings, depiction's of humans at their best.

Boredom is probably the most limiting factor to fasting a long time. That is because boredom is progressive, it gets worse with each slowly-passing day. But concurrently, the rate of healing is accelerating with each slowly-passing day. Every day the faster gets through does them considerably more good than the previous day. However, fasters rarely are motivated enough to overcome boredom for more than two weeks or so, unless they started the fast to solve a very serious or life-threatening condition. For this reason, basically well people should not expect to be able to fast for more than a couple of weeks every six months or year, no matter how much good a longer fast might do.

Exercise While Fasting

The issue of how much activity is called for on a fast is controversial. Natural Hygienists in the Herbert Shelton tradition insist that all fasters absolutely must have complete bed rest, with no books, no TV, no visitors, no enemas, no exercise, no music, and of course no food, not even a cup of herb tea. In my many years of conducting people through fasts, I have yet to meet an individual that could mentally tolerate this degree of nothingness. It is too drastic a withdrawal from all the stimulation people are used to in the twentieth century. I still don't know how Shelton managed to make his patients do it, but my guess is that he must have been a very intimidating guy. Shelton was a body builder of some renown in his day. I bet Shelton's patients kept a few books and magazines under their mattress and only took them out when he wasn't looking. If I had tried to enforced this type of sensory deprivation, I know my patients would have grabbed their clothes and run, vowing never to fast again. I think it is most important that people fast, and that they feel so good about the experience that they want to do it again, and talk all their sick friends into doing the same thing.

In contrast to enforced inactivity, Russian researchers who supervised schizophrenics on 30 day water fasts insisted that they walk for three hours every day, without stopping. I would like to have been there to see how they managed to enforce that. I suspect some patients cheated. I lived with schizophrenics enough years to know that it is very difficult to get them to do anything that they don't want to do, and very few of them are into exercise, especially when fasting.

In my experience both of these approaches to activity during the fast are extremes. The correct activity level should be arrived at on an individual basis. I have had clients who walked six miles a day during an extended water fast, but they were not feeling very sick when they started the fast, and they were also physically fit. In contrast I have had people on extended fasts who were unable to walk for exercise, or so weak they were unable to even walk to the bathroom, but these people were critically ill when they started fasting, and desperately needed to conserve what little vital force they had for healing.

Most people who are not critically ill need to walk at least 200 yards twice a day, with assistance if necessary, if only to move the lymph through the system. The lymphatic system is a network of ducts and nodes which are distributed throughout the body, with high concentrations of nodes in the neck, chest, arm pits, and groin. Its job is to carry waste products from the extremities to the center of the body where they can be eliminated. The blood is circulated through the arteries and veins in the body by the contractions of the heart, but the lymphatic system does not have a pump. Lymphatic fluid is moved by the contractions of the muscles, primarily those of the arms and legs. If the faster is too weak to move, massage and assisted movements are essential.

Lymph nodes are also a part of our immune system and produce white blood cells to help control invading organisms. When the lymph is overloaded with waste products the ducts and nodes swell, and until the source of the local irritation is removed, are incapable of handling further debris. If left in this condition for years they become so hard they feel like rocks under the skin. Lumps in the armpits or the groin are prime sites for the future development of a cancer. Fasting, massage, and poultices will often soften overloaded lymph nodes and coax them back into operation.

The Stages *of* Fasting

The best way to understand what happens when we fast is to break up the process into six stages: preparation for the fast, loss of hunger, acidosis, normalization, healing, and breaking the fast.

A person that has consumed the typical American diet most of their life and whose life is not in immediate danger would be very wise to gently prepare their body for the fast. Two weeks would be a minimum amount of time, and if the prospective faster wants an easier time of it, they should allow a month or even two for preliminary housecleaning. During this time, eliminate all meat, fish, dairy products, eggs, coffee, black tea, salt, sugar, alcohol, drugs, cigarettes, and greasy foods. This de-addiction will make the process of fasting much more pleasant, and is strongly recommended. However, eliminating all these harmful substances is withdrawal from addictive substances and will not be easy for most. I have more to say about this later when I talk about allergies and addictions.

The second stage, psychological hunger, usually is felt as an intense desire for food. This passes within three or four days of not eating anything. Psychological hunger usually begins with the first missed meal. If the faster seems to be losing their resolve, I have them drink unlimited quantities of good-tasting herb teas, (sweetened–only if absolutely necessary–with nutrisweet). Salt-free broths made from meatless instant powder (obtainable at the health food store) can also fend off the desire to eat until the stage of hunger has passed.

Acidosis, the third stage, usually begins a couple of days after the last meal and lasts about one week. During acidosis the body vigorously throws off acid waste products. Most people starting a fast begin with an overly acid blood pH from the typical American diet that contains a predominance of acid-forming foods. Switching over to burning fat for fuel triggers the release of even more acidic substances. Acidosis is usually accompanied by fatigue, blurred vision, and possibly dizziness. The breath smells very bad, the tongue is coated with bad-tasting dryish mucus, and the urine may be concentrated and foul unless a good deal of water is taken daily. Two to three quarts a day is a reasonable amount.

Mild states of acidosis are a common occurrence. While sleeping after the last meal of the day is digested bodies normally work very hard trying to detoxify from yesterday's abuses. So people routinely awaken in a state of acidosis. Their tongue is coated, their breath foul and they feel poorly. They end their brief overnight fast with breakfast, bringing the detoxification process to a screeching halt and feel much better. Many people think they awaken hungry and don't feel well until they eat. They confuse acidosis with hunger when most have never experienced real hunger in their entire lives. If you typically awaken in acidosis, you are being given a strong sign by your body that it would like to continue fasting far beyond breakfast. In fact, it probably would enjoy fasting long beyond the end of acidosis.

Most fasters feel much more comfortable by the end of the first seven to ten days, when they enter the normalization phase; here the acidic blood chemistry is gradually corrected. This sets the stage for serious healing of body tissues and organs. Normalization may take one or two more weeks depending on how badly the body was out of balance. As the blood chemistry steadily approaches perfection, the faster usually feels an increasing sense of well-being, broken by short spells of discomfort that are usually healing crises or retracings.

The next stage, accelerated healing, can take one or many weeks more, again depending on how badly the body has been damaged. Healing proceeds rapidly after the blood chemistry has been stabilized, the person is usually in a state of profound rest and the maximum amount of vital force can be directed toward repair and regeneration of tissues. This is a miraculous time when tumors are metabolized as food for the body, when arthritic deposits dissolve, when scar tissues tend to disappear, when damaged organs regain lost function (if they can). Seriously ill people who never fast long enough to get into this stage (usually it takes about ten days to two weeks of water fasting to seriously begin healing) never find out what fasting can really do for them.

Breaking the fast is equally or more important a stage than the fast itself. It is the most dangerous time in the entire fast. If you stop fasting prematurely, that is, before the body has completed detoxification and healing, expect the body to reject food when you try to make it eat, even if you introduce foods very gradually. The faster, the spiritual being running the body, may have become bored and want some action, but the faster's body hasn't finished. The body wants to continue healing.

By rejection, I mean that food may not digest, may feel like a stone in your stomach, make you feel terrible. If that happens and if, despite that clear signal you refuse to return to fasting, you should go on a juice diet, take as little as possible, sip it slowly (almost chew it) and stay on juice until you find yourself digesting it easily. Then and only then, reintroduce a little solid raw food like a green salad.

Weaning yourself back on to food should last just as long as the fast. Your first tentative meals should be dilute, raw juices. After several days of slowly building up to solid raw fruit, small amounts of raw vegetable foods should be added. If it has been a long fast, say over three weeks, this reintroduction should be done gingerly over a few weeks. If this stage is poorly managed or ignored you may become acutely ill, and for someone who started fasting while dangerously ill, loss of self control and impulsive eating could prove fatal. Even for those fasting to cure non-life-threatening illnesses it is pointless to go through the effort and discipline of a long fast without carefully establishing a correct diet after the fast ends, or the effort will have largely been wasted.

Foods *for* Monodiet, Juice *or* Broth Fasting

zucchini, garlic, onion, green beans, kale, celery, beet greens and root, cabbage, carrot, wheat grass juice, alfalfa juice, barley green juice, parsley juice, lemon/lime juice, grapefruit juice, apples (not juice, too sweet), diluted orange juice, diluted grape juice

Less-Rigorous-Than-Water Fasts

There are gradations of fasting measures ranging from rigorous to relatively casual. Water fasting is the most rapid and effective one. Other methods have been created by grasping the underlying truth of fasting, namely whenever the digestive effort can be reduced, by whatever degree, whenever the formation of the toxins of misdigestion can be reduced or prevented, to that extent the body can divert energy to the healing process. Thus comes about assorted famous and sometimes notorious monodiet semi-fasts like the grape cure where the faster eats only grapes for a month or so, or the lemon cure, where the juice of one or more lemons is added to water and nothing else is consumed for weeks on end. Here I should also mention the "lemon juice/cayenne pepper/maple syrup cure," the various green drink cures using spirulina, chlorella, barley green or wheat grass, and the famous Bieler broths–vegetable soups made of overcooked green beans or zucchini.

I do not believe that monodiets work because of some magical property of a particular food used. They work because they are semi-fasts and may be extremely useful, especially for those individuals who cannot or will not tolerate a water fast.

The best foods for monodiet fasting are the easiest ones to digest: juices of raw fruits and nonstarchy vegetables with all solids strained out. Strained mineral broths made of long-simmered non-starchy vegetables (the best of them made of leafy green vegetables) fall in the same category. So if you are highly partial to the flavor of grapes or lemons or cayenne and (highly diluted) maple syrup, a long fast on one of these would do you a world of good, just not quite as much good as the same amount of time spent on water alone. If you select something more "solid" for a long monodiet fast, like pureed zucchini, it is essential that you not overeat. Dr. Bieler gave his fasting patients only one pint of zucchini soup three or four times a day. The way to evaluate how much to eat is by how much weight you are losing. When fasting, you must lose weight! And the faster the better.

Pure absolute water fasting while not taking any vitamins or other nutritional supplementation has a very limited maximum duration, perhaps 45 days. The key concept here is nutritional reserves. Body fat is stored, surplus energy fuel. But energy alone cannot keep a body going. It needs much more than fuel to rebuild and repair and maintain its systems. So the body in its wisdom also stores up vitamins and minerals and other essential substances in and in-between all its cells. Bodies that have been very well nourished for a long time have very large reserves; poorly nourished ones may have very little set aside for a rainy day. And it is almost a truism that a sick person has, for quite some time, been a poorly nourished one. With low nutritional reserves. This fact alone can make it difficult for a sick person to water fast for enough time to completely heal their damaged organs and other systems.

Obese people have fat reserves sufficient to provide energy for long periods, but rarely can anybody, no matter how complete its nutrition was for years previously, contain sufficient nutritional reserves to support a water fast of over six weeks. To water fast the very obese down to normal weight can take months but to make this possible, rather diverse and concentrated nutrition containing few calories must be given. It is possible to fast even a very slim a person for quite a bit longer than a month when their body is receiving easily assimilable vitamins and minerals and small amounts of sugars or other simple carbohydrates.

I estimate that fasting on raw juices and mineral broths will result in healing at 25 to 75 percent of the efficiency of water fasting, depending on the amount of nutrition taken and the amount the juices or broths are diluted. But juice fasting can permit healing to go on several times longer than water might.

Fasting on dilute juice and broth can also save the life of someone whose organs of elimination are insufficiently strong to withstand the work load created by water fasting. In this sense, juices can be regarded as similar to the moderators in a nuclear reactor, slowing the process down so it won't destroy the container. On a fast of undiluted juice, the healing power drops considerably, but a person on this regimen, if not sick, is usually capable of working.

Duration of juice fasts can vary greatly. Most of the time there is no need to continue fasting after the symptoms causing concern have been eliminated, and this could happen as quickly as one week or take as long as 60 days if the person is very obese. Fasters also lose their motivation once the complaint has vanished. But feeling better is no certain indication that the need to fast has ended. This points up one of the liabilities of juice fasting; the person is already eating, their digestive system never shut down and consequently, it is much easier for them to resume eating. The thing to keep in mind is that if the symptoms return, the fast was not long enough or the diet was not properly reformed after the fast.

During a long fast on water or dilute juice, if the body has used up all of it's reserves and/or the body has reached skeletal condition, and the condition or symptoms being addressed persists the fast should be ended, the person should go on a raw food healing diet. If three to six months on raw food don't solve the complaint then another spell of water or dilute juice fasting should be attempted. Most fasters are incapable of persisting until the body reserves have been used up because social conditioning is telling them their emaciated-looking body must be dying when it is actually far from death, but return of true hunger is the critical indicator that must not be ignored. True hunger is not what most people think of when they think they are hungry. Few Americans have ever experienced true hunger. It is not a rumbling in the stomach or a set of uncomfortable sensations (caused by the beginning of detoxification) you know will go away after eating. True hunger is an animal, instinctual feeling in the back of one's throat (not in the stomach) that demands you eat something, anything, even grass or shoe leather.

Seriously ill people inevitably start the cleansing process with a pre-existing and serious mineral deficiencies. I say inevitably because they likely would not have become ill had they been properly nourished. Sick fasters may be wise to take in minerals from thin vegetable broths or vitamin-like supplements in order to prevent uncomfortable deficiency states. For example calcium or magnesium deficiencies can make water fasters experience unpleasant symptoms such as hand tremors, stiff muscles, cramps in the hands, feet, and legs, and difficulty relaxing. I want to stress here that fasting itself does not create deficiencies. But a person already deficient in minerals should watch for these symptoms and take steps to remedy the deficiencies if necessary.

Raw Food Healing Diets

Next in declining order of healing effectiveness is what I call a raw food healing diet or cleansing diet. It consists of those very same watery fruits and nonstarchy vegetables one juices or makes into vegetable broths, but eaten whole and raw. Heating food does two harmful things: it destroys many vitamins, enzymes and other nutritional elements and it makes many foods much harder to digest. So no cooked vegetables or fruits are allowed because to maintain health on this limited regimen it is essential that every possible vitamin and enzyme present in the food be available for digestion. Even though still raw, no starchy or fatty vegetables or fruits are allowed that contain concentrated calories like potatoes, winter squash, avocados, sweet potatoes, fresh raw corn, dates, figs, raisins, or bananas. And naturally, no salad dressings containing vegetable oils or (raw) ground seeds are allowed. Nor are raw grains or other raw concentrated energy sources.

When a person starts this diet they will at first experience considerable weight loss because it is difficult to extract a large number of calories from these foods (though I have seen people actually gain weight on a pure melon diet, so much sugar do these fruits have, and well-chewed watermelon seeds are very nourishing). Eating even large quantities of only raw fruit and raw non-starchy vegetables results in a slow but steady healing process about 10 to 20 percent as rapid as water fasting.

A raw food cleansing diet has several huge advantages. It is possible to maintain this regimen and regularly do non-strenuous work for many months, even a year or more without experiencing massive weight loss and, more important to some people, without suffering the extremes of low blood sugar, weakness and loss of ability to concentrate that happen when water fasting. Someone on a raw food cleanse will have periods of lowered energy and strong cravings for more concentrated foods, but if they have the self-discipline to not break their cleansing process they can accomplish a great deal of healing while still maintaining more or less normal (though slower paced) life activities. However, almost no one on this diet is able to sustain an extremely active life-style involving hard physical labor or competitive sports. And from the very beginning someone on a raw food cleanse must be willing and able to lie down and rest any time they feel tired or unable to face their responsibilities. Otherwise they will inevitably succumb to the mental certainty that their feelings of exhaustion or overwhelm can be immediately solved by eating some concentrated food to "give them energy." Such low-energy states will, however, pass quickly after a brief nap or rest.

Something else gradually happens to a body when on such a diet. Do you recall that I mentioned that after my own long fast I began to get more "mileage" out of my food. A cleansed, healed body becomes far more efficient at digestion and assimilation; a body that is kept on a raw food cleansing diet will initially lose weight rapidly, but eventually weight loss slows to virtually nothing and then stabilizes. However, long-term raw fooders are usually thin as toothpicks.

Once starchy vegetables like potatoes or winter squash, raw or cooked, or any cereals, raw or cooked, are added to a cleansing diet, the detoxification and healing virtually ceases and it becomes very easy to maintain or even gain weight, particularly if larger quantities of more concentrated foods like seeds and nuts are eaten. Though this diet has ceased to be cleansing, few if any toxins from misdigestion will be produced and health is easy to maintain.

"Raw fooders" are usually people who have healed themselves of a serious diseases and ever after continue to maintain themselves on unfired food, almost as a matter of religious belief. They have become convinced that eating only raw, unfired food is the key to extraordinarily long life and supreme good health. When raw fooders wish to perform hard physical work or strenuous exercise, they'll consume raw nuts and some raw grains such as finely-ground oats soaked overnight in warm water or deliciously sweet "Essene bread," made from slightly sprouted wheat that is then ground wet, made into cakes, and sun baked at temperatures below about 115 degrees Fahrenheit. Essene bread can be purchased in some health food stores. However, little or no healing or detoxification can happen once concentrated energy sources are added to the diet, even raw ones.

During my days at Great Oaks School I was a raw fooder for some years, though I found it very difficult to maintain body heat on raw food during chilly, rainy Oregon winters and eventually struck a personal compromise where I ate about half my diet raw and the rest fired. I have listed some books by raw fooders in the Bibliography. Joe Alexander's is the most fun.

Complete Recovery *of the* Seriously Ill

It's a virtual certainty that to fully recover, a seriously ill person will have to significantly rebuild numerous organs. They have a hard choice: to accept a life of misery, one that the medical doctors with drugs and surgery may be able to prolong into an interminable hell on earth, or, spend several years working on really healing their body, rotating between water fasting, juice or broth fasting, extended periods on a cleansing raw food diet, and periods of no-cleansing on a more complete diet that includes moderate amounts of cooked vegetables and small quantities of cooked cereals. And even after recovery someone who was quite ill may have to live the rest of their life on a rather restricted regimen.

It is unrealistic to expect one fast to fix everything. The body will heal as much as it can in the allotted time, but if a dangerous illness has not been fully remedied by the first intense fast, a raw food diet must be followed for three to six months until weight has been regained, nutritional reserves have been rebuilt and it is safe to undertake another extended fast. More than two water or juice fasts a year of thirty continuous days are not recommended nor should they be necessary unless the life is in imminent danger and there is no other option.

The story of Jake's catastrophic illness and almost-cure is a good example of this type of program. Jake was from back East. He phoned me because he had read a health magazine article I had written, his weak voice faintly describing a desperate condition. He was in a wheelchair unable to walk, unable to control his legs or arms very well, was unable to control his bladder and required a catheter. He had poor bowel control, had not the strength to talk much or loudly and most frightening to him, he was steadily losing weight although he was eating large amounts of cooked vegetables and grains. Jake had wasted away to 90 pounds at 5' 10" and looked pathetic when I first saw him wheeled off an airplane at my local airport.

Jake had seen a lot of medical doctors and had variously been diagnosed as having chronic fatigue syndrome, chronic (whatever that is) meningitis, and multiple sclerosis. He had been treated by virtually every medical expert and many famous alternative practitioners, utilizing a host of old and new techniques, all to no avail. He had even tried intravenous chelation therapy and colonics. It had also been suggested that he enter a hospital for the treatment of eating disorders and/or see a psychiatrist. He had tried to gain admittance to a number of holistic fasting institutions back east, but they all refused him because they considered the risk was too high to fast a person at such a low body weight. But I had previously fasted emaciated people like Jake, and there was something I liked about his telephone presence. Perhaps this is why I foolishly decided I knew better than the other experts.

People commonly waste away and die while eating large amounts of food. Obviously they are unable to digest or assimilate nutrients or they wouldn't be wasting. Eating further increases their toxic burden from undigested meals, further worsening their already failing organs. The real solution is to stop feeding them altogether so that their digestive functions can heal. In Jake's case, his body's nutritional reserves had already become sadly depleted due to poor absorption over such an extended period, so I could not fast him on water. I immediately put Jake on a rich mineral broth prepared from everything left alive in our garden at the end of winter–leaves of kale, endive plants, whole huge splitting Savoy cabbages, garlic, huge leeks including their green tops, the whole stew fortified with sea weed. It did not matter too much what vegetables I used as long as there were lots of leafy greens containing lots of chlorophyll (where the most concentrated mineral nutrition is located).

Jake was given colonics every day, but had to be carried to the colonic table because he could not support his own weight. Whoever had given him colonics previously had not accomplished much for I must say that Jake had the most foul smelling discharges that I had ever encountered in administering over 6,000 colonics over many years. It was as if his body was literally rotting from the inside out.

After 30 days on mineral broth Jake, who really did weigh 90 pounds when he arrived, was only down to 85! When a person already close to skeletal weight starts fasting, to conserve vital tissue the body goes rapidly into a state of profound rest so it uses very little energy, thus it loses very little weight each day. This degree of resting also helps heal abnormal body parts earlier. After one month on mineral broth Jake began to show signs of mineral deficiencies in the form of a fine tremor of the hands, and cramps in the feet, so I put him on mineral supplements too.

Jake was in my house for a long time. At the end of the second month on broth he started two weeks on raw carrot juice with a lot of chlorophyll added from sources such as algae (spirulina), wheat grass juice, alfalfa, etc.. This was followed by two more weeks on small quantities of raw fruits and vegetables, and then followed by two weeks with added steamed vegetables, and finally, he achieved a diet which included small amounts of grain, cooked legumes and raw nuts, plus the fruits and vegetables previously mentioned. Jake health steadily improved. He gained control of his bladder, bowels, speech, hands, and legs. He began to exercise in the living room on a stationary bike, and walked slowly up and down our long driveway, picking daffodils in the beautiful spring weather.

Sadly, though I could help his body to heal it was next to impossible to stem the tides of Jake's appetites or to pleasantly withstand his tantrums when he was denied; he always wanted more in terms of quantity, more in terms of variety, and at more frequent intervals. Though his organs had healed significantly, his digestive capacity was not nearly as large as he remembered himself enjoying before he got sick. And never would be. Jake was not happy about the dietary restrictions necessary for him to retain his newly attained health, and unwilling to stay within the limits of his digestive system's ability to process foods. He had gained weight and was back up to 120 pounds. It was time for him to go home before I lost my good humor.

Jake left with a lot of "good lucks" and stern admonitions to stick to his stringent diet and supplement program. It was a big moment for Jake. He had arrived in a wheelchair three months before. Now he walked unaided to the airplane, something he had not been able to do for two years.

Back at home Jake had no one courageous enough to set limits for him. His immediate family and every one of his brow beaten associates were compelled to give him everything that he wanted. So his appetite and lack of personal discipline got the better of him. He started eating lots of dates and figs. These had been eliminated from his diet because he was unable to process foods which such a high sugar content. He also ate larger and larger quantities of grains, nuts and avocados, although I had warned him of specific quantity limits on rich foods. Most sadly, he returned to enjoying spaghetti with lots of cheese grated on top. Within months of leaving my care his paralysis and weakness returned, except that unfortunately for him, he still retained the ability to assimilate food and maintain his body weight. Ironically, the only ultimate benefit of his fasting with me was to permit him to suffer a far longer existence in a wheelchair without wasting away and escaping into death.

I would be failing my readers if I did not explain why Jake became ill in the first place. Jake had started what grew to become a very successful chain of spaghetti restaurants with a unique noodles and sauces made to his own formula. He ate a lot of his own spaghetti over the years, and had been reared in a good Italian family with lots of other kinds of rich food. Jake had a reputation for being able to outeat everybody in terms of quantity and in the amount of time spent eating. In childhood, this ability had made his Italian mother very happy because it showed appreciation for her great culinary skill.

Secondly, Jake the adult was still at his core, Jake the spoiled brat child, with a bad, unregulated temper. He was in the habit of dumping his temper on other people whether they needed a helping of his angry emotions or not. A lot of people in his employ and in his extended family tiptoed around Jake, always careful of triggering his wrath. At my place as Jake began to get well he began to use his increased energy and much stronger voice to demonstrate his poor character. At meal times Jake would bang the table with a fork hard enough to leave dents in the wood table top while yelling for more, complaining loudly about the lack of rich sauces and other culinary delights he craved. This was a character problem that Jake could not seem to overcome, even with a lot of intervention from the local minister on his behalf and my counseling. Jake was a Catholic who went to church regularly, but acted like a Christian only while he was in church. On some level Jake knew that he was not treating others fairly, but he would not change his habitual responses. His negative thoughts and actions interfered with his digestive capacity to the extent that his gluttonous eating habits produced illness, a vegetative paralyzing illness, but not death. To me this seems almost a form of karmic justice.

It is common for people who have been very ill for extended periods of time to realize what a wonderful gift life is and arrive at a willingness to do almost anything to have a second chance at doing "life" right. Some succeed with their second chance and some don't. If they don't succeed in changing their life and relationships, they frequently relapse.

Luigi Cornaro's left the world his story of sickness and rejuvenation. His little book may be the world's first alternative healing text. It is a classic example of the value of abstentousness. Had Jake taken this story to heart he would have totally recovered. Cornaro was a sixteenth century Venetian nobleman. He, like Jake the spaghetti baron, was near death at the young age of forty. (Jake was also in his early 40s when he broke down.) Cornaro's many doctors were unable to cure him. Finally he saw a doctor who understood the principles of natural healing. This wise physician determined that this illness was caused by a mismatch between Cornaro's limited digestive capacity and the excessive amount of food he was eating. So Cornaro was put on a diet of only 12 ounces of solid food and fourteen ounces of liquid a day. Any twelve ounces of any solids he wanted and any fourteen ounces of liquid. It could be meat and wine, salad or orange juice, no matter.

Cornaro soon regained his health and he continued to follow the diet until the age of 78. His health was so outstanding during this period that people who were much younger in terms of years were unable to keep up with him. At 78 his friends, worried about how thin he was (doesn't it always seem that it is your so-called friends who always ruin a natural cure) persuaded him to increase his daily ration by two ounces a day. His delicate and weak digestive system, which had operated perfectly for many years, was unable to deal with the additional two ounces, and he became very ill after a very short period of over eating.

Worse, his recent indulgence had even further damaged the organs of digestion and to survive Cornaro had to cut his daily ration to eight ounces of solid food and eleven of liquids. On this reduced dietary he again regained his health and lived to be 100. Cornaro wrote four books on the value of abstinence or "sober living" as he called it, writing the last and perhaps the most interesting at 96 years of age. Had my patient Jake been able to confine his food intake to the level of his body's ability to digest, he might still be walking and enjoying life. But try as I might I could not make him understand. Perhaps he enjoys doing penance in his wheel chair more than he would enjoy health and life.

Tissue Losses at Death *by* Starvation

Fat	97%
Muscles	31
Blood	27
Liver	54
Spleen	67
Pancreas	17
Skin	21
Intestines	18
Kidneys	26
Lungs	18
Testes	40
Heart	3
Brain and Spinal Cord	3
Nerves	3
Bone	14

From Keys, Ancel, Joseph Brozek, Austin Henchel, Olaf Mickelson and Henry L. Taylor, (1950) *The Biology of Human Starvation*. Two Vols. Minneapolis: University of Minnesota Press.

Starvation

It is true that ethical medical doctors use the least-risky procedure they are allowed to use. But this does not mean there are no risks to allopathic treatment. The medical doctor justifies taking the risks by saying that the risk/reward ratio is the best possible. Any sick person is already at risk. Life comes with only one guarantee: that none of us gets out of it alive.

Compared to the risks of allopathic medicine, fasting is a far safer method of treating disease. The oft-repeated scare stories medical doctors and their allies circulate about fasting are not true, and it is important to remember that none of these people portraying fasting as evil and dangerous have ever fasted themselves–I'll put money on that one. Or, on the slim possibility that someone telling fasting horror stories did actually not eat for 24 hours (probably because some accident or acute illness prevented them), they had a terrible experience because they didn't understand the process, were highly toxic, and were scared to death the whole time.

Or worse yet they fasted for a short period with an "open mind"–a very dangerous state in which to approach anything new. I have found through considerable experience with people professing to have open minds that the expression "I'm open minded" usually means that someone has already made up their mind and new data just passes straight through their open mind–in one ear and out the other. Or sometimes, the phrase "open mind" means a person that does not believe any information has reality and is entirely unable to make up their mind.

The most commonly leveled criticism of fasting is that in its efforts to survive self-imposed starvation the body metabolizes vital tissue, not just fat, and therefore, fasting is damaging, potentially fatally damaging. People who tell you this will also tell you that fasters have destroyed their heart muscle or ruined their nervous system permanently. But this kind of damage happen only when a person starves to death or starves to a point very close to death, not when someone fasts.

There is a huge difference between fasting and starvation. Someone starving is usually eating, but eating poorly and inadequately, eating scraps of whatever is available such as sugar, white flour, rancid grease, shoe leather, or even dirt. Frequently a starving person is forced to exercise a great deal as they struggle to survive and additionally is highly apprehensive. Or someone starving to death is confined to a small space, may become severely dehydrated too and is in terror. Fear is very damaging to the digestive process, and to the body in general; fear speeds up the destruction of vital tissue. People starve when trekking vast distances through wastelands without food to eat, they starved in concentration camps, buried in mind disasters, they starve during famines and starve while being tortured in prisons.

Until water fasting goes on past the point where all fatty tissues and all abnormal deposits have been burned for fuel and recycled for the nutritional elements they contain, vital muscle tissues and organs are not consumed. And as long as the body contains sufficient nutritional reserves, vital organs and essential tissues are rebuilt and maintained. In fact the body has a great deal of intelligence that we don't give it credit for. It knows exactly which cells are essential to survival, which ones are not. The body knows which cells are abnormal deposits, and it goes to work to metabolize them first. For example, the body recognizes arthritic deposits, cysts, fibroids, and tumors as offensive parts of the landscape, and obligingly uses them for foods in preference to anything else. A starving (not fasting) body also knows precisely in what order of priority body cells should be metabolized to minimize risk of death or permanent disability.

After a starving body has reached skeletal condition, or where some small amount of fat remains but nutritional reserves (vitamins and minerals) are exhausted and there is insufficient nourishment forthcoming, the body begins to consume nutrient-rich muscle and organ tissue in a last-ditch effort to stay alive. Under these dire circumstances, the least essential muscles and organs from the standpoint of survival are metabolized first. For example, muscles in the arms and legs would be consumed early in the process, the heart muscle used only toward the very end. The very last part of the body to be metabolized when one is starving and as has come very close to death would be the brain and the nervous system.

Starvation begins where fasting ends, which is when real hunger begins. If the return of hunger is ignored whenever it takes place, whether it is in 30, 60, or 90 days depending upon body weight and type of fast, at that point exactly, not a day before, starvation begins very slowly. Usually it takes a considerable period of time after that before death occurs. It is important to note that this discussion applies only to the abstention from food, not water. Death takes place very quickly in the absence of water.

The chart on the previous page shows numerically the phenomenal ability of the body to protect the most essential tissues of the body right up to the time of death. If a person fasted for 30 days, the average time it takes for the return of hunger in a person that is not overweight, and then ignored the return of hunger, and continued to abstain from food–if the person could avoid forced exercise, keep warm, and had enough hydration, it could take as much as an additional 20 to 60 days to die of starvation! At death the body would have experienced losses of 40 to 60 percent of its starting body weight. (Ancel Keys et al, 1950) A emaciated person cannot afford to lose nearly as much weight as an obese person, and death under conditions of starvation will occur earlier. In all cases of starvation the brain, nerves, heart, lungs, kidneys and liver remain largely intact and functional to the very end. During a fast, it is almost impossible to damage essential organs, unless of course the person creates the damage by fears about the process, or by internalizing the fears of others. If those fears are present, the fast should not be attempted.

Weight Loss *by* Fasting

Loss of weight indicates, almost guarantees, that detoxification and healing is occurring. I can't stress this too much. Of all the things I find my patients seem to misunderstand or forget after being told, it is that they can't heal in a rapid manner without getting smaller. This reality is especially hard for the family and friends of someone who is fasting, who will say, "you're looking terrible dear, so thin. Your skin is hanging on your bones. You're not eating enough protein or nutrient food to be healthy and you must eat more or you're going to develop serious deficiencies. You don't have any energy, you must be getting sicker. You're doing the wrong thing, obviously. You have less energy and look worse every day. Go and see a doctor before it is too late." To succeed with friends like this, a faster has to be a mighty self-determined person with a powerful ability to disagree with others.

Medical personnel claim that rapid weight loss often causes dangerous deficiencies; these deficiencies force the person to overeat and regain even more weight afterward. This is largely untrue, though there is one true aspect to it: a fasted, detoxified body becomes a much more efficient digester and assimilator, extracting a lot more nutrition from the same amount food is used to eat. If, after extended fasting a person returns to eating the same number of calories as they did before; they will gain weight even more rapidly than before they stated fasting. When fasting for weight loss, the only way to keep the weight off is to greatly reform the diet; to go on, and stay on, a diet made up largely of non-starchy, watery fruits and vegetables, limited quantities of cooked food, and very limited amounts of highly concentrated food sources like cereals and cooked legumes. Unless, of course, after fasting, one's lifestyle involves much very hard physical labor or exercise. I've had a few obese fasters become quite angry with me for this reason; they hoped to get thin through fasting and after the fast, to resume overeating with complete irresponsibility as before, without weight gain.

People also fear weight loss during fasting because they fear becoming anorexic or bulimic. They won't! A person who abstains from eating for the purpose of improving their health, in order to prevent or treat illness, or even one who fasts for weight loss will not develop an eating disorder. Eating disorders mean eating compulsively because of a distorted body image. Anorexics and bulimics have obsessions with the thinner-is-better school of thought. The anorexic looks at their emaciated frame in the mirror and thinks they are fat! This is the distorted perception of a very insecure person badly in need of therapy. A bulimic, on the other hand stuffs themselves, usually with bad food, and then purges it by vomiting, or with laxatives. Anorexics and bulimics are not accelerating the healing potential of their bodies; these are life threatening conditions. Fasters are genuinely trying to enhance their survival potential.

Occasionally a neurotic individual with a pre-existing eating disorder will become obsessed with fasting and colon cleansing as a justification to legitimize their compulsion. During my career while monitoring hundreds of fasters, I've known two of these. I discourage them from fasting or colon cleansing, and refuse to assist them, because they carry the practices to absurd extremes, and contribute to bad press about natural medicine by ending up in the emergency ward of a hospital with an intravenous feeding tube in their arm.

Cases Beyond The Remedy Of Fasting

Occasionally, very ill people have a liver that has become so degenerated it cannot sustain the burden of detoxification. This organ is as vital to survival as the brain, heart and lungs. We can get along with only one kidney, we can live with no spleen, with no gallbladder, with only small parts of the stomach and intestines, but we cannot survive without a liver for more than a day or so. The liver is the most active organ in the body during detoxification. To reach an understanding of detoxification, it helps to know just what the liver does for us on an ongoing basis.

The liver is a powerful chemical filter where blood is refined and purified. The liver passes this cleansed blood out through the superior vena cava, directly to the heart. The blood is then pumped into general and systemic circulation, where it reaches all parts of the body, delivering nutrition and oxygen at a cellular level. On its return flow, a large proportion of the depleted blood is collected by the gastric, splenic and superior and inferior mesenteric veins that converge to form the large portal vein which enters the liver. Thus a massive flow of waste from all the cells of the body is constantly flowing into the liver. The huge hepatic artery also enters the liver to supply oxygen and nutrients with which to sustain the liver cells themselves.

The liver is constantly at work refining the blood. It is synthesizing, purifying, renovating, washing, filtering, separating, and detoxifying. It works day and night without stopping. Many toxins are broken down by enzymes and their component parts are efficiently reused in various parts of the body. Some impurities are filtered out and held back from the general circulation. These debris are collected and stored in the gall bladder, which is a little sack appended to the liver. After a meal, the contents of the gall bladder (bile) are discharged into the duodenum, the upper part of the small intestine just beyond the stomach. This bile also contains digestive enzymes produced by the liver that permit the breakdown of fatty foods in the small intestine.

Sometimes a large flow of bile finds its way into the stomach by pressure or is sucked into the stomach by vomiting. Excessive biliary secretion and excretion can also result from overeating, which overcrowds the area. Sometimes colonics or massage can also stimulate a massive flow of bile. Extremely bitter and irritating, when bile gets into the stomach the person either vomits or wishes they could. And after vomiting and experiencing the taste of bile, wishes they hadn't.

When no food at all enters the system, the blood keeps right on passing through the liver/filter just as it does when we are eating. When the liver does not have to take care of toxins generated by the current food intake, each passage through the liver results in a cleaner blood stream, with the debris decreasing in quantity, viscosity, and toxicity, until the blood becomes normalized. During fasting, debris from the gall bladder still pass through the small intestine and into the large intestine. However, if the bowels do not move the toxins in the bile are readsorbed into the blood stream and get recirculated in an endless loop. This toxic recycling makes a faster feel just terrible, like they had a flu or worse!

The bowels rarely move while fasting. During fasting only enemas or colonics permit elimination from the large intestine. If done effectively and frequently, enemas will greatly add to the well being and comfort of the faster. Many times when a faster seems to be retracing or experiencing a sudden onset of acute discomfort or symptoms, these can be almost immediately relieved by an enema or colonic.

A person with major liver degeneration inevitably dies, with or without fasting, with or without traditional medicine. Significantly impaired kidney function can also bring about this same result. Mercifully, death while fasting is usually accomplished relatively free of pain, clear of mind and with dignity. That often cannot be said of death in a hospital. There are much worse experiences than death.

Fasting is not a cure-all. There are some conditions that are beyond the ability of the body to heal. Ultimately, old age gets us all.

Dr. Linda Hazzard, one of the greats of natural hygiene, who practiced Osteopathic medicine in the 1920s, had a useful way of categorizing conditions that respond well to fasting. These she labeled "acute conditions," and "chronic degenerative conditions." A third classification, "chronic conditions with organic damage," does not respond to fasting. Acute conditions, are usually inflammations or infections with irritated tissue, with swelling, redness, and often copious secretions of mucous and pus, such as colds, flu, a first time case of pneumonia, inflamed joints as in the early stages of arthritis, etc. These acute conditions usually remedy in one to three weeks of fasting. Acute conditions are excellent candidates for self-doctoring. Chronic degenerative conditions are more serious and the patient usually requires supervision. These include conditions such as cancer, aids, chronic arthritis, chronic pneumonia, emphysema and asthma. Chronic degenerative conditions usually respond within a month to three months of fasting. The fasting should be broken up into two or three sessions if the condition has not been relieved in one stint of supervised fasting. Each successive fast will produce some improvement and if a light, largely raw-food diet is adhered to between fasts the patient should not worsen and should be fairly comfortable between fastings.

If there has been major functional damage to an organ as a result of any of these degenerative conditions, healing will not be complete, or may be impossible. By organic damage, I mean that a vital part of the body has ceased to function due to some degenerative process, injury, or surgery–so badly damaged that the cells that make up the organ cannot be replaced.

I once had a twenty five year old man come to my spa to die in peace because he had been through enough diagnostic procedures in three hospitals to know that his liver was beyond repair. He had been working on an apple farm in between terms at university when he was poisoned several times with insecticide from an aerial spray on the whole orchard. He absorbed so much insecticide that his liver incurred massive organic damage.

When he came to me his body had reached the point where it was incapable of digesting, and because of lack of liver function, it was incapable of healing while fasting, a condition in which death is a certainty. He was a Buddhist, did not fear death and did not want to be kept alive in agony or in prolonged unconsciousness by any extraordinary means, nor did he want to die with tubes in every orifice. I was honored to be a supportive participant in his passing. He died fasting, in peace, and without pain, with a clear mind that allowed him to consciously prepare for the experience. He was not in a state of denial or fear, and made no frantic attempts to escape the inevitable. He went quietly into that still dark night with a tranquil demeanor and a slight smile.

Fortunately, in my many years of practice I had the pleasure of seeing the majority of the people totally regain their health or at least greatly improve it by means of the fasting and healing diets. Many cancer patients watched with amazement as their tumors disappeared before their eyes, many arthritics regained their function, serious skin conditions such as psoriasis disappeared, mental conditions improved, addictions vanished, fatigue was replaced by energy, and fat dissolved revealing the hidden sculpture beneath. I will talk more about procedures and the particular reasons bodies develop specific conditions in later chapters.

Social/Cultural/Psychological Obstacles *to* Fasting

Numerous attitudes make it difficult to fast or to provide moral support to friends or loved ones that are fasting. Many people harbor fears of losing weight because they think that if times were really tough, if there was a famine or they became ill and lost a lot of weight they would have no reserves and would certainly perish. These people have no idea how much fat can be concealed on an even skinny body, nor of how slowly a skinny body loses weight while fasting. Substantial fat reserves are helpful as heat-retaining insulation in those rare accidents when someone is dropped into a cold ocean and must survive until the rescue boat arrives. Being fat might keep a person alive longer who is lost in the wilderness awaiting rescue with no supplies, no means of procuring food, and no means of keeping warm. On the other hand, fat people would have a far harder time walking out of the wilderness. And extensive fat deposits are merely fuel and do not contain extensive nutritional reserves. An obese person fasting without significant nutritional supplementation would begin starving long before they became really skinny. On the balance, carrying excess weight is a far greater liability than any potential prosurvival aspects it might have.

There are other attitudes associated with weight loss that make it difficult for people to fast. People hold rather stereotypical notions about what constitutes an attractive person; usually it involves having some meat on ones bones. Hollywood and Hugh Hefner have both influenced the masses to think that women should have hourglass figures with large, upthrust, firm breasts. Since breasts are almost all useless fatty tissue supporting some milk-producing glands that do not give a breast much volume except when engorged, most women fasters loose a good percentage of their breast mass. If the fast is extensive, there should also develop an impressive showing of ribs and hip bones; these are not soft and cuddly. Husbands, lovers, parents, and friends frequently point out that you don't look good this way and exhort you to put on weight. Most people think pleasantly plump is healthy.

Skinny men, especially those who had lost a lot of weight during an illness, are pressured by associates to put on weight to prove that they are healthy. I had a client who was formerly a college varsity football player. Before his illness he had lifted weights and looked like a hunk. His family and friends liked to see him that way and justifiably so. Then he got seriously ill. On a long extended healing diet he lost a significant amount of weight and seemed downright skinny, causing all who knew him well and cared about him to tempt him with all kinds of scrumptious delicacies from the best of kitchens. But this case was like Luigi Cornaro, a man who never again could look like a hunk. His "friends" made an absolutely necessary change in life style and appearance far more difficult than it was already. My client was torn between a desire to please others, and a desire to regain and retain his health. This problem a sick person doesn't need.

If you have the independence to consider following an alternative medical program in a culture that highly values conformity and agreement, you are also going to have to defend your own course of self-determined action based on the best available data that you have. But fasters are usually in fragile emotional condition, so I advise my clients who are subjected to this kind of pressure to beg their friends and associates to refrain from saying anything if they can't support the course of action you have chosen. After this, if friends or relatives are still incapable of saying nothing (even non-verbally), it is important to exclude them from your life until you have accomplished your health goals, have regained some weight and have returned to eating a maintenance diet, rather than getting skinnier on a healing one.

The very worst aspect of our culture's eating programming is that people have been wrongfully taught that when ill they must eat to keep up their strength. Inherent in this recommendation is an unstated belief that when the body is weakened by a disease state, the weakness can somehow be overcome with food, and that the body needs this food to kill the virus, bacteria, or invading yeast, and uses the protein to heal or rebuild tissue. Sadly, the exact opposite is the case. Disease organisms feed and multiply on the toxic waste products of misdigestion, and the body is unable to digest well when it is weak or ill.

There's an old saying about this: "feed a cold, starve a fever." Most people think this saying means you should eat when you have a cold. What the saying really means is if you feed a cold then you will soon have to starve a fever. Protein foods especially are not digested by a diseased body, and as mentioned before, the waste products of protein indigestion are especially poisonous. That is all the body needs when it is already down, another load of poison which it can't eliminate due to weakness and enervation.

Weight loss is usually associated with illness, as it should be! In times of acute illness an otherwise healthy body loses its appetite for food because it is prosurvival to stop eating. It is very hard to coax a sick animal to eat. Their bodies, not controlled by a mind full of complex learned responses and false ideas, automatically know that fasting is nature's method of healing. Contrary to popular understanding, digestion, assimilation, and elimination require the expenditure of considerable energy. This fact may contradict the reader's experience because everyone has become tired when they have worked a long time without eating, and then experienced the lift after eating. But an ill body cannot digest efficiently so instead of providing energy extracted from foods, the body is further burdened by yet another load of toxic material produced by fermented and putrefied food. This adds insult to injury in a sick body that is already drowning in its own garbage.

Worse, during illness most available vital force is already redirected into healing; it is not available for digestion. It is important to allow a sick body to proceed with healing and not to obstruct the process with unnecessary digestion or suppress the symptoms (which actually are the healing efforts) with drugs. If you have an acute illness, and you stop all food intake except for pure water and herb teas, and perhaps some vegetable broth, or dilute non-sweet juice, you have relieved your body of an immense effort. Instead of digesting, the body goes to work on catching up on healing. The body can and will almost inevitably heal itself if the sick person will have faith in it, cooperate with the body's efforts by allowing the symptoms of healing to exist, reduce or eliminate the intake of food to allow the body to marshal its energies, maintain a positive mental attitude and otherwise stay out of the way.

Many people intensely dread missing even one meal. These folks usually are and have been so toxic that their bodies had been stashing uneliminated toxins in their fat for years. They are usually so addicted to caffeine, cigarettes, alcohol, and so forth, that when they had fasted, even briefly, their bodies were forced to dip into highly-polluted fat reserves while simultaneously the body begins withdrawal. People like this who try to fast experience highly unpleasant symptoms including headache, irritability, inability to think or concentrate, blurred vision, profound fatigue, aches, etc. Most of these symptoms come from low blood sugar, but combined with the toxins being released from fat and combined with going through multiple addictive withdrawals, the discomforts are more than most people are willing to tolerate. Fasting on juice is much more realistic for cases like this. It is little wonder that when a hygienist suggests a fast to improve health, this type of case asserts positively that fasting is quite impossible, they have tried it, it is absolutely terrible and know that they can't do it.

This rejection is partly due to a cultural expectation (one reinforced by western medicine) that all unpleasant symptoms should be avoided or suppressed. To voluntarily experience unpleasant sensations such as those mentioned above is more than the ordinary timid person will subject themselves to, even in order to regain health. They will allow surgery, drugs with violent and dangerous side effects, painful and invasive testing procedures and radiation—all unpleasant and sometimes extremely uncomfortable. These therapies are accepted because someone else with authority is doing it to them. And, they have been told that it they don't submit they will not ever feel better and probably will die in the near future. Also people think that they have no alternative, that the expert in front of them knows what is best, so they feel relieved to have been relieved of the responsibility for their own condition and its treatment.

Preventative Fasting

During the years it takes for a body to degenerate enough to prompt a fast, the body has been storing up large quantities of unprocessed toxins in the cells, tissues, fat deposits, and organs. The body in its wisdom will always choose to temporarily deposit overwhelming amounts of toxins somewhere harmless rather than permit the blood supply to become polluted or to use secondary elimination routes. A body will use times when the liver is less burdened to eliminate these stored toxic debris. The hygienists' paradigm asserts that the manifestation of symptoms or illness are all by themselves, absolute, unassailable proof that further storage of toxic wastes in the cells, tissues, fat deposits, and organs is not possible and that an effort toward elimination is absolutely necessary. Thus the first time a person fasts a great quantity of toxins will normally be released. Being the resident of a body when this is happening can be quite uncomfortable. For this reason alone, preventative fasting is a very wise idea.

Before the body becomes critically ill, clean up your reserve fuel supply (fat deposits) by burning off some accumulated fat that is rich in toxic deposits and then replace it with clean, non-toxic fat that you will make while eating sensibly. If you had but fasted prophylactically as a preventative or health-creating measure before you became seriously ill, the initial detoxification of your body could have been accomplished far more comfortably, while you were healthy, while your vital force was high and while your body otherwise more able to deal with detoxification.

Each time you fast, even if it is only one day, you allow your body to go through a partial detox, and each time it becomes easier and more comfortable than the last time. The body learns how to fast. Each time you fast it, your body slips into a cleansing mode more quickly, and each time you fast you lighten the load of stored toxins. Perhaps you have already eliminated the caffeine your body had stored, which frequently causes severe headaches on withdrawal, not to mention fatigue. It certainly helps to have this behind you before you go on to the elimination of other irritating substances. Many people have gone through alcohol or tobacco withdrawal, and understand that it is very unpleasant, and also that it must be done in the pursuit of health. Why not withdraw from the rest of the irritating and debilitating substances we take into our system on an ongoing basis, and why not grit your way through the eliminative process, withdraw, from food addictions such as sugar or salt, and from foods that you may be allergic to like wheat, dairy products or eggs.

It is very wise to invest in your own insurance plan by systematically detoxifying while you are still healthy. Plan it into your life, when it is convenient, such as once a week on Sunday, or even once a month on a quiet day. Take a few days of vacation, go to a warm, beautiful place and devote part or all of it to cleansing. Treat yourself by taking an annual trip to Hawaii, fasting at a hotel on the beach–do whatever it takes to motivate yourself. And consider this: vacations are enormously cheaper when you stay out of restaurants.

If you have accustomed your body to 24 hour fasts, then you can work on 48 hour fasts, and over time work up to 72 hour fasts, all on a continuum. You may find it becoming increasingly comfortable, perhaps even pleasant, something you look forward to. Fasting a relatively detoxified body feels good, and people eventually really get into the clean, light, clear headed, perhaps spiritually aware state that goes along with it.

By contrast, fasting when you are sick is much more difficult because your vitality or vital force is very low, you already have no energy, and probably have unpleasant symptoms that must be dealt with at the same time. There may be the added stress of being forced into a cleanse because you are too nauseous to eat. Most people let their health go until they are forced into dealing with it; they are too busy living, so why bother.

The truth is that our body does age, and over time becomes less able to deal with insults; the accumulated effect of insults and aging eventually leads most of us to some serious degenerative illness. Normally this begins happening around age 50 if not sooner. Some of us that were gifted with good genes or what I call "a good start" may have reached the age of 60 or 75 or even 90 without serious illness, but those people are few and far between. Why not tip the scales in your favor by preventing or staving off health problems with systematic detoxification at your own convenience.

Climb into the driver's seat and start to take control and gain confidence in your own ability to deal with your body, your own health, and your own life. When it gets right down to the bottom line, there is really only one thing in the world that is really yours, and that is your life. Take control and start managing it. The reward will be a more qualitative life.

Chapter Four

Colon Cleansing

From The Hygienic Dictionary

Autointoxication. [1] the accumulations on the bowel wall become a breeding ground for unhealthy bacterial life forms. The heavy mucus coating in the colon thickens and becomes a host for putrefaction. The blood capillaries to the colon begin to pick up the toxins, poisons and noxious debris as it seeps through the bowel wall. All tissues and organs of the body are now taking on toxic substances. Here is the beginning of true autointoxication on a physiological level. *Bernard Jensen, Tissue Cleansing Through Bowel Management.* [2] All maladies are due to the lack of certain food principles, such as mineral salts or vitamins, or to the absence of the normal defenses of the body, such as the natural protective flora. When this occurs, toxic bacteria invade the lower alimentary canal, and the poisons thus generated pollute the bloodstream and gradually deteriorate and destroy every tissue, gland and organ of the body. *Sir Arbuthnot Lane.* [3] The common cause of gastro-intestinal indigestion is enervation and overeating When food is not digested, it becomes a poison. Dr. John H. Tilden, Impaired Health: Its Cause and Cure, 1921. [4] a clogging up of the large intestine by a building up (on) the bowel wall to such an extent that feces can hardly pass through. autointoxication is a direct result of intestinal constipation. Faulty nutrition is a major underlying factor in constipation. The frequency or quantity of fecal elimination is not an indication of the lack of constipation in the bowel.
Bernard Jensen, Tissue Cleansing Through Bowel Management.

I am not a true believer in any single healing method or system. I find much truth in many schools and use a wide variety of techniques. The word for my inclination is eclectic.

The most effective medicine in my arsenal is water fasting followed closely in potency by other, less rigorous detoxifying diets. Colon cleansing ranks next in healing power. In fact it is difficult to separate colon cleansing from fasting because detoxification programs should always be accompanied by colon cleansing. Further down the scale of efficatiousness comes dietary reform to eliminate allergic reactions and to present the body with foods it is capable of digesting without creating toxemia. Last, and usually least in effectiveness in my arsenal, are orthotropic substances (in the form of little pills and capsules) commonly known as vitamins or food supplements.

Interestingly, acceptance of these methods by my clients runs in exact opposition to their effectiveness. People prefer taking vitamins because they seem like the allopaths' pills, taking pills demands little or no responsibility for change. The least popular prescription I can write is a monodiet of water for several weeks or a month. Yet this is my most powerful medicine.

It is possible to resolve many health complaints without fasting, simply by cleansing the colon and regaining normal lower bowel function. Colonics take little personal effort and are much easier to get people to accept than fasting. So I can fully understand how perfectly honest and ethical naturopaths have developed obsessions with colon cleansing. Some healers have loudly and repeatedly (and wrongly) proclaimed that constipation is the sole cause of disease, and thus, the only real cure for any illness is colon cleansing.

Even though it is possible to have a lot of successes with the simple (though unpleasant to administer) technique of colon cleansing, degenerated lower bowels are the only cause of disease. I prefer to use bowel cleansing as an adjunct to more complete healing programs. However, old classics of hygiene and even a few new books strongly make the case for colonics. Some of these books are entirely one-sided, single-cause single-cure approaches, and sound convincing to the layperson. For this reason, I think I should take a few paragraphs and explain why some otherwise well-intentioned health professionals have overly-advocated colonics (and other practices as well).

Most Diseases Cure Themselves

If you ask any honest medical doctor how they cure diseases, they will tell you that most acute disease conditions and a smaller, though significant percentage (probably a majority) of chronic disease conditions are self-limiting and will, given time, get better all by themselves. So for most complaints, the honest allopathic doctor sees their job as giving comfort and easing the severity of the symptoms until a cure happens.

This same scenario, when viewed from a hygienist's perspective, is that almost all acute and many chronic conditions are simply the body's attempt to handle a crisis of toxemia. For two reasons the current crisis will probably go away by itself. The positive reason is that the toxic overload will be resolved: the person changes their dietary habits or the stressor that temporarily lowered their vital force and produced enervation is removed, then digestion improves and the level of self-generated toxins is reduced. The negative reason for a complaint to "cure" itself is that the suffering person's vital force drops below the level that the symptom can be manifested and the complaint goes away because a new, more serious disease is developing.

I view this second possibility as highly undesirable because strong, healthy bodies possessing a high degree of vital force are able to eliminate toxins rather violently, frequently producing very uncomfortable symptoms that are not life-threatening. However, as the vital force drops, the body changes its routes of secondary elimination and begins using more centrally located vital organs and systems to dispose of toxemia. This degeneration producing less unpleasant symptoms, but in the long run, damages essential organs and moves the person closer to their final disease.

A young vigorous body possessing a large degree of vital force will almost always route surplus toxins through skin tissues and skin-like mucus membranes, producing repeated bouts of sinusitis, or asthma, or colds, or a combination of all these. Each acute manifestation will "cure" itself by itself eventually. But eventually the body's vital force can no longer create these aggressive cleansing phenomena and the toxemia begins to go deeper. When the allopathic doctor gets a patient complaining of sinusitis, they know they will eventually get a cure. The "cure" however, might well be a case of arthritis.

This unfortunate reality tends to make young, idealistic physicians become rather disillusioned about treating degenerative conditions because the end result of all their efforts is, in the end, death anyway. The best they can do is to alleviate suffering and to a degree, prolong life. The worst they can do is to prolong suffering.

Thus, the physicians main job is to get the patient to be patient, to wait until the body corrects itself and stops manifesting the undesired symptom. Thus comes the prime rule of all humane medicine: first of all, do no harm! If the doctor simply refrains from making the body worse, it will probably get better by itself. But the patient, rarely resigned to quiet suffering, comes in demanding fast relief, demanding a cure. In fact, if the patient were resigned to quiet suffering they would not consult a doctor. So if the doctor wants to keep this patient and make a living they must do something. If that something the doctor must do does little or no harm and better yet, can also alleviate the symptoms, the doctor is practicing good medicine and will have a very high cure rate and be financially successful if they have a good bedside manner. This kind of doctor may be allopathic and/or "natural," may use herbs or practice homeopathy.

The story of Dr. Jennings, a very successful and famous or infamous (depending on your viewpoint) physician, who practiced in Connecticut in the early 1800s exemplifies this type of approach.

Dr. Jennings had his own unique medicines. Their composition was of his own devising, and were absolutely secret. He had pills and colored bitter drops of various sorts that were compounded himself in his own pharmacy. Dr. Jennings' patients generally recovered and had few or no complications. This must be viewed in contrast to the practices of his fellow doctors of that era, whose black bags were full of mercury and arsenic and strychnine, whose practices included obligatory bleeding. These techniques and medicines "worked" by poisoning the body or by reducing its blood supply and thus lowering its vital force, ending the body's ability to manifest the undesirable symptom. If the poor patient survived being victimized by their own physician, they were tough enough to survive both their disease and the doctor's cure. Typically, the sick had many, lengthy complications, long illnesses, and many "setbacks" requiring many visits, earning the physician a great living.

Dr. Jennings operated differently. He would prescribe one or two secret medicines from his black bag and instruct the patient to stay in bed, get lots of rest, drink lots of water, eat little and lightly, and continue taking the medicine until they were well. His cure rate was phenomenal. Demand they might, but Dr. Jennings would never reveal what was in his pills and vials. Finally at the end of his career, to instruct his fellow man, Dr. Jennings confessed. His pills were made from flour dough, various bitter but harmless herbal substances, and a little sugar. His red and green and black tinctures, prescribed five or ten drips at a time mixed in a glass of water several times daily, were only water and alcohol, some colorant and something bitter tasting, but harmless. Placebos in other words.

Upon confessing, Dr. Jennings had to run for his life. I believe he ended up retiring on the western frontier, in Indiana. Some of his former patients were extremely angry because they had paid good money, top dollar for "real" medicines, but were given only flour and water. The fact that they got better didn't seem to count.

If the physicians curative procedure suppresses the symptom and/or lowers the vital force with toxic drugs or surgery, (either result will often as not end the complaint) the allopathic doctor is practicing bad medicine. This doctor too will have a high cure rate and a good business (if they have an effective bedside manner) because their drugs really do make the current symptoms vanish very rapidly. Additionally, their practice harmonizes with a common but vicious dramatization of many people which goes: when a body is malfunctioning, it is a bad body and needs to be punished. So lets punish it with poisons and if that don't work, lets really punish it by cutting out the offending part.

However, if the physician can do something that will do no harm but raises the vital force and/or lowers the level of toxemia, this doctor will have a genuine cure rate higher than either of the two techniques. Why does raising the vital force help? Because it reduces enervation, improves the digestion, lowers the creation of new toxins and improves the function of the organs of elimination, also reducing the toxic overload that is causing the complaint.

Techniques that temporarily and quickly raise the vital force include homeopathy, chiropractic, vitamin therapy, massage, acupuncture and acupressure and many more spiritually oriented practices. Healers who use these approaches and have a good bedside manner can have a very good business, they can have an especially-profitable practice if they do nothing to lower the level of toxemia being currently generated. Their patients do experience prompt relief but must repeatedly take the remedy. This makes for satisfied customers and a repeat business.

The best approach of all focuses on reducing the self-generated level of toxemia, cleansing to remove deposits of old toxemia, rebuilding the organs of elimination and digestion to prevent the formation of new toxemia, and then, to alleviate the current symptoms and make it easier for the patient to be patient while their body heals, the healer raises artificially and temporarily the vital force with vitamins, massage, acupressure, etc. This wise and benevolent physician is going to have the highest cure rate among those wise patients who will accept the prescription, but will not make as much money because the patients permanently get better and no longer need a physician. There's not nearly as much repeat business.

Colonics are one of the best types of medicine. They clean up deposits of old toxemia (though there are sure to be other deposits in the body's tissues colonics do not touch). Colon cleansing reduces the formation of new toxemia from putrefying fecal matter (but dietary reform is necessary to maximize this benefit). Most noticeable to the patient, a colonic immediately alleviates current symptoms by almost instantly reducing the current toxic load. A well-done enema or colonic is such a powerful technique that a single one will often make a severe headache vanish, make an onsetting cold go away, end a bout of sinusitis, end an asthmatic attack, reduce the pain of acute arthritic inflammation, reduce or stop an allergic reaction. Enemas are also thrifty: they are self-administered and can prevent most doctor's visits seeking relief for acute conditions.

Diseases of the colon itself, including chronic constipation, colitis, diverticulitis, hemorrhoids, irritable bowel syndrome, and mucous colitis, are often cured solely by an intensive series of several dozen colonics given close together. Contrary to popular belief, many people think that if they have dysentery or other forms of loose stools that a colonic is the last thing they need. Surprisingly, a series of colonics will eliminate many of these conditions as well. People with chronic diarrhea or loose stools are usually very badly constipated. This may seem a contradiction in terms but it will be explained shortly.

A century ago there was much less scientific data about the functioning of the human body. Then it was easy for a hygienically-oriented physician to come to believe that colonics were the single best medicine available. The doctor practicing nothing but colonics will have a very high rate of cure and a lot of very satisfied clients. Most importantly, this medicine will have done no harm.

The Repugnant Bowel

I don't know why, but people of our culture have a deep-seated reluctance to relate to the colon or its functions. People don't want to think about the colon or personally get involved with it by giving themselves enemas or colonics. They become deeply embarrassed at having someone else do it for them. People are also shy about farts, and most Americans have a hard time not smiling or reacting in some way when someone in their presence breaks wind, although the polite amongst us pretend that we didn't notice. Comedians usually succeed in getting a laugh out of an audience when they come up with a fart or make reference to some other bowel function. People don't react the same way to urinary functions or discharges, although these also may have an unpleasant odor and originate from the same "private" area.

When I first mention to clients that they need a minimum of 12 colonics or many more enemas than 12 during a fasting or cleansing program they are inevitably shocked. To most it seems that no one in their right mind would recommend such a treatment, and that I must certainly be motivated by greed or some kind of a psychological quirk. Then I routinely show them reproductions of X-rays of the large intestine showing obvious loss of normal structure and function resulting from a combination of constipation, the effects of gravity, poor abdominal muscle tone, emotional stress, and poor diet. In the average colon more than 50% of the hastrum (muscles that impel fecal matter through the organ) are dysfunctional due to loss of tone caused by impaction of fecal matter and/or constriction of the large intestine secondary to stress (holding muscular tension in the abdominal area) and straining during bowel movement.

A typical diseased colon

The average person also has a prolapsed (sagging) transverse colon, and a distorted misplaced ascending and descending colon. I took a course in colon therapy before purchasing my first colonic machine. The chiropractor teaching the class required all of his patients scheduled for colonics to take a barium enema followed by an X-ray of their large intestine prior to having colonics and then make subsequent X-rays after each series of 12 colonics. Most of his patients experienced so much immediate relief they voluntarily took at least four complete series, or 48 colonics, before their X-rays began to look normal in terms of structure. It also took about the same number, 48 colonics, for the patients to notice a significant improvement in the function of the colon. In reviewing over 10,000 X-rays taken at his clinic prior to starting colonics, the chiropractor had seen only two normal colon X-rays and these were from farm boys who grew up eating simple foods from the garden and doing lots of hard work.

The X-rays showed that it took a minimum of 12 colon treatments to bring about a minimal but observable change in the structure of the colon in the desired direction, and for the patient to begin to notice that bowel function was improving, plus the fact that they started to feel better.

A Healthy Colon

From my point of view the most amazing part of this whole experience was that the chiropractor did not recommend any dietary changes whatsoever. His patients were achieving great success from colonics alone. I had thought dietary changes would be necessary to avoid having the same dismal bowel condition return. I still think colonics are far more effective if people are on a cleansing diet too. However, I was delighted to see the potential for helping people through colonics.

For me, the most interesting part of this colonic school was that I personally was required to have my own barium enema and X-ray. I was privately certain that mine would look normal, because after all, I had been on a raw food diet for six years, and done considerable amount of fasting, all of which was reputed to repair a civilized colon. Much to my surprise my colon looked just as mangled and dysfunctional as everyone else's, only somewhat worse because it had a loop in the descending colon similar to a cursive letter "e" which doctors call a volvulus. Surgeons like to cut volvululii out because they frequently cause bowel obstructions. It seemed quite unfair. All those other people with lousy looking colons had been eating the average American diet their whole life, but I had been so 'pure!'

On further reflection I remembered that I had a tendency toward constipation all through my childhood and young adulthood, and that during my two pregnancies the pressure of the fetus on an already constipated bowel had made it worse resulting in the distorted structure seen in the X-ray. This experience made it very clear that fasting, cleansing diets, and corrected diet would not reverse damage already done. Proper diet and fasting would however, prevent the condition of the colon from getting any worse than it already was.

I then realized that I had just purchased the very tool I needed to correct my own colon, and I was eager to get home to get started on it. I had previously thought that I was just going to use this machine for my patients, because they had been asking for this kind of an adjunct to my services for some time. I ended up giving myself over a hundred colonics at the rate of three a week over many months. I then out of curiosity had another barium enema and X-ray to validate my results. Sure enough the picture showed a colon that looked far more 'normal' with no vulvulus. That little "e" had disappeared.

What Is Constipation?

Most people think they are not constipated because they have a bowel movement almost every day, accomplished without straining. I have even had clients tell me that they have a bowel movement once a week, and they are quite certain that they are not constipated. The most surprising thing to novice fasters is that repeated enemas or colonics during fasting begins to release many pounds of undeniably real, old, caked fecal matter and/or huge mucus strings. The first-time faster can hardly believe these were present. These old fecal deposits do not come out the first time one has enemas or necessarily the fifth time. And all of them will not be removed by the tenth enema. But over the course of extended fasting or a long spell of light raw food eating with repeated daily enemas, amazing changes do begin to occur. It seems that no one who has eaten a civilized diet has escaped the formation of caked deposits lining the colon's walls, interfering with its function. This material does not respond to laxatives or casually administered enemas.

Anyone who has not actually seen (and smelled) what comes out of an "average" apparently healthy person during colonics will really believe it could happen or can accurately imagine it. Often there are dark black lumpy strings, lumps, or gravel, evil smelling discs shaped like sculpted hemispheres similar to the pockets lining the wall of the colon itself. These discs are rock-hard and may come out looking like long black braids. There may also be long tangled strings of gray/brown mucous, sheets and flakes of mucous, and worse yet, an occasional worm (tape worm) or many smaller ones. Once confronted however, it is not hard to imagine how these fecal rocks and other obnoxious debris interfere with the proper function of the colon. They make the colon's wall rigid and interfere with peristalsis thus leading to further problems with constipation, and interfere with adsorption of nutrients.

Our modern diet is by its "de-"nature, very constipating. In the trenches of the First World War, cheese was given the name 'chokem ass' because the soldiers eating this as a part of their daily ration developed severe constipation. Eaten by itself or with other whole foods, moderate amounts of cheese may not produce health problems in people who are capable of digesting dairy products. But cheese when combined with white flour becomes especially constipating. White bread or most white-flour crackers contain a lot of gluten, a very sticky wheat protein that makes the bread bind together and raise well. But white flour is lacking the bran, where most of the fiber is located. And many other processed foods are missing their fiber.

In an earlier chapter I briefly showed how digestion works by following food from the mouth to the large intestine. To fully grasp why becoming constipated is almost a certainty in our civilization a few more details are required. Food leaving the small intestine is called chyme, a semi-liquid mixture of fiber, undigested bits, indigestible bits, and the remains of digestive enzymes. Chyme is propelled through the large intestine by muscular contractions. The large intestine operates on what I dub the "chew chew train" principle, where the most recent meal you ate enters the large intestine as the caboose (the last car of a train) and helps to push out the train engine (the car at the front that toots), which in a healthy colon should represent the meal eaten perhaps twelve hours earlier. The muscles in the colon only contract when they are stretched, so it is the volume of the fecal matter stretching the large intestine that triggers the muscles to push the waste material along toward the rectum and anus.

Eating food lacking fiber greatly reduces the volume of the chyme and slows peristalsis. But moving through fast or slow, the colon still keeps on doing another of its jobs, which is to transfer the water in the chime back into the bloodstream, reducing dehydration. So the longer chime remains in the colon, the dryer and harder and stickier it gets. That's why once arrived at the "end of the tracks" fecal matter should be evacuated in a timely manner before it gets to dry and too hard to be moved easily. Some constipated people do have a bowel movement every day but are evacuating the meal eaten many days or even a week previously.

Most hygienists believe that when the colon becomes lined with hardened fecal matter it is permanently and by the very definition of the word itself, constipated. This type of constipation is not perceived as an uncomfortable or overly full feeling or a desire to have a bowel movement that won't pass. But it has insidious effects. Usually constipation delays transit time, increasing the adsorption of toxins generated from misdigestion of food; by coating and locking up significant portions of colon it also reduces the adsorption of certain minerals and electrolytes.

Sometimes, extremely constipated people have almost constant runny bowels because the colon has become so thickly and impenetrably lined with old fecal matter that it no longer removes much moisture. This condition is often misinterpreted as diarrhea. The large intestine's most important task is to transfer water-soluble minerals from digested food to the blood. When a significant part of the colon's surface becomes coated with impermeable dried rigid fecal matter or mucus it can no longer assimilate effectively and the body begins to experience partial mineral starvation in the presence of plenty. It is my observation from dozens of cases that when the colon has been effectively cleansed the person has a tendency to gain weight while eating amounts of food that before only maintained body weight, while people who could not gain weight or who were wasting away despite eating heavily begin to gain. And problems like soft fingernails, bone loss around teeth or porous bones tend to improve.

The Development *of* My Own Constipation

The history of my own constipation, though it especially relates to a very rustic childhood, is typical of many people. I was also raised on a very constipating diet which consisted largely of processed cheese and crackers. Mine was accelerated by shyness, amplified by lack of comfortable facilities.

I spent my early years on the Canadian prairies, where everybody had an outhouse. The fancy modern versions are frequently seen on construction sites. These are chemical toilets, quiet different than the ones I was raised with because somebody or something mysteriously comes along, empties them and installs toilet paper. The ones I'm familiar with quickly developed a bad-smelling steaming mound in the center–or it was winter when the outhouse was so cold that everything froze almost before it hit the ground in the hole below. (And my rear end seemed to almost freeze to the seat!) The toilet paper was usually an out of season issue of Eatons mail order catalogue with crisp glossy paper. Perhaps it is a peculiarity of the north country, but at night there are always monsters lurking along the path to the outhouse, and darkness comes early and stays late.

When nature called and it was daylight, and there was no blizzard outside, the outhouse received a visit from me. If on the other hand, when it was dark (we had no electricity), and there was a cold wind creating huge banks of snow, I would 'just skip it,' because the alternative–an indoor chamber pot, white enamel with a lid–was worse. This potty had to be used more or less publicly because the bedrooms were shared and there was no indoor bathroom. I was always very modest about my private parts and private functions, and potty's were only used in emergencies, and usually with considerable embarrassment. No one ever explained to me that it was not good for me to retain fecal matter, and I never thought about it unless my movements became so hard that it was painful to eliminate.

Later in life, I continued this pattern of putting off bowel movements, even though outhouses and potties were a thing of the past. As a young adult I could always think of something more interesting to do than sitting on a pot, besides it was messy and sometimes accompanied by embarrassing sound effects which were definitely not romantic if I was in the company of a young man. During two pregnancies the tendency to constipation was aggravated by the weight of the fetus resting on an already sluggish bowel, and the discomfort of straining to pass my first hard bowel movement after childbirth with a torn perineum I won't forget.

Rapid Relief *from* Colon Cleansing

During fasting the liver is hard at work processing toxins released from fat and other body deposits. The liver still dumps its wastes into the intestines through the bile duct. While eating normally, bile, which contains highly toxic substances, is passed through the intestines and is eliminated before too much is reabsorbed. (It is the bile that usually makes the fecal matter so dark in color.) However, reduction of food bulk reduces or completely eliminates peristalsis, thus allowing intestinal contents to sit for extended periods. And the toxins in the bile are readsorbed, forming a continuous loop, further burdening the liver.

The mucus membranes lining the colon constantly secrete lubricants to ease fecal matter through smoothly. This secretion does not stop during fasting; in fact, it may increase because intestinal mucus often becomes a secondary route of elimination. Allowed to remain in the bowel, toxic mucus is an irritant while the toxins in it may be reabsorbed, forming yet another closed loop and further burdening the liver.

Daily enemas or colonics administered during fasting or while on cleansing diets effectively remove old fecal material stored in the colon and immediately ease the livers load, immediately relieve discomfort by allowing the liver's efforts to further detoxify the blood, and speed healing. Fasters cleansing on juice or raw food should administer two or three enemas in short succession every day for the first three days to get a good start on the cleansing process, and then every other day or at very minimum, every few days. Enemas or colonics should also be taken whenever symptoms become uncomfortable, regardless of whether you have already cleaned the colon that day or not. Once the faster has experienced the relief from symptoms that usually comes from an enema they become more than willing to repeat this mildly unpleasant experience.

Occasionally enemas, by filling the colon and making it press on the liver, induce discharges of highly toxic bile that may cause temporary nausea. Despite the induced nausea it is still far better to continue with colonics because of the great relief experienced after the treatment. If nausea exists or persists during colon cleansing, consider trying slight modifications such as less or no massage of the colon in the area of the gall bladder (abdominal area close to the bottom of the right rib cage), and putting slightly less water in the colon when filling it up. It also helps to make sure that the stomach is empty of any fluid for one hour prior to the colonic. Resume drinking after the colonic sessions is completed. If you are one of these rare people who 'toss their bile', just keep a plastic bucket handy and some water to rinse out the mouth after, and carry on as usual.

Enemas *versus* Colonics

People frequently wonder what is the difference between a colonic and an enema.

First of all enemas are a lot cheaper because you give them to yourself; an enema bag usually costs about ten dollars, is available at any large drug store, and is indefinitely reusable. Colonics cost anywhere from 30 to 75 dollars a session.

Chiropractors and naturopaths who offer this service hire a colonic technician that may or may not be a skilled operator. It is a good idea to find a person who has a very agreeable and professional manner, who can make you feel at ease since relaxation is very important. It is also beneficial to have a colonic therapist who massages the abdomen and foot reflexes appropriately during the session.

Enemas and colonics can accomplish exactly the same beneficial work. But colonics accomplish more improvement in less time than enemas for several reasons. During a colonic from 30 to 50 gallons of water are flushed through the large intestines, usually in a repetitive series of fill-ups followed by flushing with a continuous flow of water. This efficiency cannot even be approached with an enema. But by repeating the enema three times in close succession a satisfactory cleanse can be achieved. Persisted with long enough, enemas will clean the colon every bit as well as a colonic machine can.

Enemas given at home take a lot less time than traveling to receive a colonics at someone's clinic, and can be done entirely at you own convenience—a great advantage when fasting because you can save your energy for internal healing. But colonics are more appropriate for some. There are fasters who are unable to give themselves an enema either because their arms are too short and their body is too long and they lack flexibility, or because of a physical handicap or they can't confront their colon, so they let someone else do it. Some don't have the motivation to give themselves a little discomfort but are comfortable with someone else doing it to them. Some very sick people are too weak to cleanse their own colon, so they should find someone to assist them with an at-home enema or have someone take them to a colonic therapist.

Few people these days have any idea how to properly give themselves an enema. The practice has been discredited by traditional medical doctors as slightly dangerous, perhaps addictive and a sign of psychological weirdness. Yet Northamericans on their civilized, low fiber, poorly combined diets suffer widely from constipation. One proof of this is the fact that chemical laxatives, with their own set of dangers and liabilities, occupy many feet of drug store shelf space and are widely advertised. Is the medical profession's disapproval of the enema related to the fact that once the initial purchase of an enema bag has been made there are no further expenses for laxatives? Or perhaps it might be that once a person discovers they can cure a headache, stop a cold dead in its tracks with an enema, they aren't visiting the M.D.s so often.

The enema has also been wrongly accused of causing a gradual loss of colon muscle tone, eventually preventing bowel movements without the stimulation of an enema, leading finally to flaccidity and enlargement of the lower bowel. This actually can happen; when it does occur it is the result of frequent administration of small amounts of water (fleet enemas) for the purpose of stimulating a normal bowel movement. The result is constant stretching of the rectum without sufficient fluid to enter the descending colon. A completely opposite, highly positive effect comes from properly administered enemas while cleansing.

The difference between helpful and potentially harmful enemas lies in the amount of water injected and the frequency of use. Using a cup or two of water to induce a bowel movement may eventually cause dependency, will not strengthen the colon and may after years of this practice, result in distention and enlargement of the rectum or sigmoid colon. However, a completely empty average-sized colon has the capacity of about a gallon of water. When increasingly larger enemas are administered until the colon is nearly emptied of fecal matter and the injection of close to a gallon of water is achieved, beneficial exercise and an increase in overall muscle tone are the results.

Correctly given, enemas (and especially colonics) serve as strengthening exercises for the colon. This long tubular muscle is repeatedly and completely filled with water, inducing it to vigorously exercise while evacuating itself multiple times. The result is a great increase in muscle tone, acceleration of peristalsis and eventually, after several dozens of repetitions, a considerable reduction of transit time. Well-done enemas work the colon somewhat less effectively and do not improve muscle tone quite as much as colonics.

Injecting an entire gallon of water with an enema bag is very impractical when a person is eating normally. But on a light cleansing diet or while fasting the amount of new material passing into the colon is small or negligible. During the first few days of fasting if two or three enemas are administered each day in immediate succession the colon is soon completely emptied of recently eaten food and it becomes progressively easier to introduce larger amounts of water. Within a few days of this regimen, injecting half a gallon or more of water is easy and painless.

Probably for psychological reasons, some peoples' colons allow water to be injected one time but then "freeze up" and resist successive enemas. For this reason better results are often obtained by having one enema, waiting a half hour, another enema, wait a half hour, and have a final enema.

A colonic machine in the hands of an expert operator can administer the equivalent of six or seven big enemas in less than one hour, and do this without undue discomfort or effort from the person receiving the colonic. However, the AMA has suppressed the use of colonics; they are illegal to administer in many states. Where colonics are legal, the chiropractors now consider this practice messy and not very profitable compared to manipulations. So it is not easy to find a skilled and willing colonic technician.

Anyone who plans to give themselves therapeutic enemas while fasting would be well advised to first seek out a colonic therapist and receive two or three colonics delivered one day apart while eating lightly and then immediately begin the fast. Three colonics given on three successive days of a light, raw food diet are sufficient to empty all recently eaten food even from a very constipated, distended and bloated colon, while acquainting a person with their own bowel. Having an empty colon is actually a pleasant and to most people a thoroughly novel experience. A few well-delivered colonics can quickly accustom a person to the sensations accompanying the enema and demonstrate the effect to be achieved by oneself with an enema bag, something not quickly discoverable any other way.

How To Give Yourself An Enema

Enemas have been medically out of favor for a long time. Most people have never had one. So here are simple directions to self-administer an effective enema series.

The enema bag you select is important. It must hold at least two quarts and be rapidly refillable. The best American-made brand is made of rubber with about five feet of rubber hose ending in one of two different white hard plastic insertion tips. The bag is designed for either enemas or vaginal douches. It hangs from a detachable plastic "S" hook. When filled to the brim it holds exactly one-half gallon. The maker of this bag offers another model that costs about a dollar more and also functions as a hot water bottle. A good comforter it may make, but the dual purpose construction makes the bag very awkward to rapidly refill. I recommend the inexpensive model.

The plastic insertion tips vary somewhat. The straight tubular tip is intended for enemas; the flared vaginal douche tip can be useful for enemas too, in that it somewhat restrains unintentional expulsion of the nozzle while filling the colon. However, its four small holes do not allow a very rapid rate of flow.

To give yourself an enema, completely fill the bag with tepid water that does not exceed body temperature. The rectum is surprisingly sensitive to heat and you will flinch at temperatures only a degree or two higher than 98 Fahrenheit. Cooler water is no problem; some find the cold stimulating and invigorating. Fasters having difficulty staying warm should be wary of cold water enemas. These can drop core body temperature below the point of comfort.

Make sure the flow clamp on the tube is tightly shut and located a few inches up the tube from the nozzle. Hang the filled bag from a clothes or towel hook, shower nozzle, curtain rod, or other convenient spot about four to five feet above the bathroom floor or tub bottom. The higher the bag the greater the water pressure and speed of filling. But too much pressure can also be uncomfortable. You may have to experiment a bit with this.

Various body positions are possible for filling the colon. None is correct or necessarily more effective than another. Experiment and find the one you prefer. Some fill their colon kneeling and bending forward in the bathtub or shower because there will likely be small dribbles of water leaking from around the nozzle. Usually these leaks do not contain fecal matter. Others prefer to use the bathroom floor. For the bony, a little padding in the form of a folded towel under knees and elbows may make the process more comfortable. You may kneel and bend over while placing your elbows or hands on the floor, reach behind yourself and insert the nozzle. You may also lie on your back or on your side. Some think the left side is preferable because the colon attaches to the rectum on the left side of the body, ascends up the left side of the abdomen to a line almost as high as the solar plexus, then transverses the body to the right side where it descends again on the right almost to the groin. The small intestine attaches to the colon near its lower-right extremity. In fact these are the correct names given for the parts of the colon: Ascending, Descending and Transverse Colon along with the Sigmoid Colon or Rectum at the exit end.

As you become more expert at filling your colon with water you will begin to become aware of its location by the weight, pressure and sometimes temperature of the water you're injecting. You will come to know how much of the colon has been filled by feel. You will also become aware of peristalsis as the water is evacuated vigorously and discover that sensations from a colon hard at work, though a bit uncomfortable, are not necessarily pain.

Insertion of the nozzle is sometimes eased with a little lubricant. A bit of soap or KY jelly is commonly used. If the nozzle can be inserted without lubricant it will have less tendency to slip out. However, do not tear or damage the anus by avoiding necessary lubrication. After insertion, grip the clamp with one hand and open it. The flow rate can be controlled with this clamp. Keeping a hand on the clamp also prevents the nozzle from being expelled.

Water will begin flowing into the colon. Your goal is to empty the entire bag into the colon before sensations of pressure or urgency to evacuate the water force you to remove the nozzle and head for the toilet. Relaxation of mind and body helps achieve this. You are very unlikely to achieve a half-gallon fill up on the first attempt. If painful pressure is experienced try closing the clamp for a moment to allow the water to begin working its way around the obstacle. Or, next time try hanging the bag lower, reducing its height above the body and thus lowering the water pressure. Or, try opening the clamp only partially. Or, try panting hard, so as to make the abdomen move rapidly in and out, sort of shaking the colon. This last technique is particularly good to get the water past a blockage of intestinal gas.

It is especially important for Americans, whose culture does not teach one to be tolerant of discomfort, to keep in mind that pain is the body's warning that actual damage is being done to tissues. Enemas can do no damage and pose no risk except to that rare individual with weak spots in the colon's wall from cancers. When an enema is momentarily perceived unpleasantly, the correct name for the experience is a sensation, not pain. You may have to work at increasing your tolerance for unpleasant sensations or it will take you a long time to achieve the goal of totally filling the colon with water. Be brave! And relax. A wise philosopher once said that it is a rough Universe in which only the tigers survive–and sometimes they have a hard time.

Eventually it will be time to remove the nozzle and evacuate the water. Either a blockage (usually fecal matter, an air bubble, or a tight 'U' turn in the colon, usually at either the splenetic, or hepatic flexures located right below the rib cage) will prevent further inflow (undesirable) or else the bag will completely empty (good!) or the sensation of bursting will no longer be tolerable. Go sit on the toilet and wait until all the water has passed. Then refill the bag and repeat the process. Each time you fill the colon it will allow more water to enter more easily with less unpleasantness. Fasters and cleansers should make at least three attempts at a complete fill-up each time they do an enema session.

Water and juice fasters will find that after the first few enemas, it will become very easy to inject the entire half-gallon of water. That is because there is little or no chime entering the colon. After a few days the entire colon will seem (this is incorrect) to be empty except when it is filled with water. This is the point to learn an advanced self-administered enema technique. An average colon empty of new food will usually hold about one gallon of water. That is average. A small colon might only hold 3/4 gallon, a large one might accept a gallon and a half, or even more. You'll need to learn to simultaneously refill the bag while injecting water, so as to achieve a complete irrigation of the whole colon. There are several possible methods. You might try placing a pitcher or half-gallon mason jar of tepid water next to the bag and after the bag has emptied the first time, stand up while holding the tube in the anus, refill the bag and then lie down again and continue filling. You might have an assistant do this for you. You might try hanging the bag from the shower head and direct a slow, continuous dribble of lukewarm water from the shower into the bag while you kneel or lie relaxed in the tub. This way the bag will never empty and you stop filling only when you feel fullness and pressure all the way back to the beginning of the ascending colon. Of course, hanging from a slowly running shower head the bag will probably overflow and you will get splashed and so will the bathroom floor when your wet body moves rapidly from the tub to the toilet. I've imagined making an enema bag from a two gallon plastic bucket with a small plastic hose barb glued into a hole drilled in the bottom or lower edge. If I were in the business of manufacturing enema bags I'd make them hold at least one gallon.

A word of caution to those folks who have a pattern of overdoing it, or tend to think that more is better. This is not true when it comes to colon cleansing. Do not make more than three attempts to fill and clean the colon with an enema bag. Usually the colon begins to protest and won't accept any more fill-ups. When having colonics on a colonic machine it is a good idea to continue until the water comes back reasonably clear for that session. It is not a good idea for a faster to have colonics that last more than three-quarters of an hour to an hour maximum, or it will be too tiring. Even non-fasters find colonics tiring. After all, the colon is basically a big muscle that has become very lazy on a low-fiber diet.

I've personally administered over five thousand colonics, taught several dozen fasters to self-administer their own and stood by while they gave themselves one until they were quite expert. In all that experience I've only seen one person have a seriously bad result. This was a suicidally depressed water faster that I (mistakenly) allowed to administer their own colonics with my machine. This person not only took daily colonics, but allowed water to flow through their colon for as long as two hours at a time. Perhaps they were trying to wash out their mind? After several weeks of this extreme excess, the faster became highly confused and disoriented due to a severe electrolyte imbalance. They had to be taken off water fasting immediately and recovered their mental clarity in a few days. The loss of blood electrolytes happened because during colonics there occurs a sort of low-grade very slow reverse osmosis.

Curing With Enemas

It is not wise to continue regular colonics or enemas once a detoxification program has been completed and you have returned to a maintenance diet. The body should be allowed its regular functioning.

But because enemas immediately lower the toxic load on the liver, I do recommend people use them for prevention of an acute illness (you feel like you are coming down with something), and for the treatment of acute illnesses such as a cold. I also like to take one if I have been away traveling for extended periods, eating carelessly. But do not fall into a pattern of bingeing on bad food, and then trying to get rid of it through colonics or laxative. This is bulimia, the eating disorder discussed earlier.

The Sheltonite capital "N" Natural capital "H" Hygienists do not recommend any colon cleansing, ever! They think that the colon will spontaneously cleanse itself on a long water fast, but my experience learned from monitoring hundreds of fasters is that it doesn't really. Herbert Shelton also considered colon cleansing enervating and therefore undesirable. Colon cleansing does use the faster's energy but on the balance, colon cleansing saves more work on the part of an overburdened liver than it uses up.

Chapter Five

Diet & Nutrition

From The Hygienic Dictionary

Food. [1] Life is a tragedy of nutrition. In food lies 99.99% of the causes of all diseases and imperfect health of any kind. *Prof. Arnold Ehret, Mucusless Diet Healing System.* [2] But elimination will never heal perfectly just so long as you fail to discontinue the supply of inside waste caused by eating and "wrong" eating. You may clean and continue to clean indefinitely, but never with complete results up to a perfect cleanliness, as long as the intake of wrong or even too much right foods, is not stopped. *Prof. Arnold Ehret, Mucusless Diet Healing System.* [3] Cooked food favors bacterial, or organized, ferment preponderance, because cooking kills the unorganized and organized ferments, and both are needed to carry on the body's digestion. Raw foods–fruits and vegetables–favor unorganized ferment digestion, because these foods carry vitamins, which are unorganized ferments–enzymes.
Dr. John. H. Tilden, Impaired Health: Its Cause and Cure, 1921.

Recently, my younger (adult) daughter asked my advice choosing between a root canal or having a bridge made. This led to a discussion of her eating habits in general. Defending her currently less-than-optimum diet against my gentle criticism, she threw me a tough riposte. "Why," she asked, when I was raised so perfectly as a child, "when I ate only Organic food until I was ten and old enough to make you send me to public school where I could eat those lousy school lunches" (her unfeeling, heartless mother home-schooled her), "why even at that young age, (before she spent her adolescent rebellion eating junk food) why at that point did I still have a mouthful of cavities?" And she did. At age ten my daughter needed about ten fillings.

This beautiful daughter of a practicing naturopath had received what, at the time, I considered virtually perfect nutrition. She suckled hugely at her mother's abundant breast until age two. During this time her mother ate a natural foods diet. After weaning my daughter got only whole grains, a little fresh goat's milk from my goat, fruits and lots of Organic vegetables. I started my spa when my daughter was about five years old and from that point she was, like it or not, a raw fooder. And all that raw food was Organic and much of it from Great Oaks School's huge vegetable garden.

For my daughter to develop cavities on this diet is reminiscent of Woody Allen's joke in his movie "Sleeper." Do you recall this one, made about 1973? The plot is a take off on Rip Van Winkle. Woody goes into the hospital for minor surgery. Unexpectedly he expires on the operating table and his body is frozen in hopes that someday he can be revived. One hundred and fifty years later he is revived.

The priceless scene I always think of takes place in his hospital room immediately after he comes to consciousness. The doctor in charge of his case is explaining to Woody what has happened. Woody refuses to believe he died and was frozen, asserting that the whole story is a put on. Woody insists that the 'doctor' is clearly an actor hired by his friends! It absolutely can't be the year 2123. 'Oh, but it really is 2123,' insists the doctor. 'And it is no put on by his friends; all his friends are long dead; Woody knows no one at all in 2123 and had better prepare himself to start a new life.'

Woody still insists it is a put on. "I had a health food store," he says, "and all my friends ate brown rice. They can't be dead!"

And my perfectly nourished daughter couldn't have developed cavities! But she did. And if she cheated on her perfect diet, bad food could not have amounted to more than two percent of her total caloric intake from birth to age ten. I was a responsible mom and I made sure she ate right! Now my daughter was demanding to know why she had tooth decay. Fortunately, I now know the answer. The answer is rather complex, but I can give a simplified explanation.

The Confusions *about* Diets *&* Foods

Like my daughter, many people of all ages are muddled about the relationship between health and diet. Their confusions have created a profitable market for health-related information. And equally, their confusions have been created by books, magazine articles, and TV news features. This avalanche of data is highly contradictory. In fact, one reason I found it hard to make myself write my own book is that I wondered if my book too would become just another part of the confusion.

Few people are willing to tolerate very much uncertainty. Rather than live with the discomfort of not knowing why, they will create an explanation or find some answer, any answer, and then ever after, assert its rightness like a shipwrecked person clings to a floating spar in a storm. This is how I explain the genesis of many contemporary food religions.

Appropriately new agey and spiritual, Macrobiotics teaches the way to perfect health is to eat like a Japanese whole foods vegetarian–the endless staple being brown rice, some cooked vegetables and seaweeds, meanwhile balancing the "yin" and "yang" of the foods. And Macrobiotics works great for a lot of people. But not all people.

Because there's next to nothing raw in the Macrobiotic diet and some people are allergic to rice, or can get allergic to rice on that diet.

Linda Clark's Diet for a Small Planet also has hundreds of thousands of dedicated followers. This system balances the proportions of essential amino acids at every, single meal and is vegetarian. This diet also works and really helps some people, but not as well as Macrobiotics in my opinion because obsessed with protein, Clark's diet contains too many hard-to-digest soy products and makes poor food combinations from the point of digestive capacity.

Then there are the raw fooders. Most of them are raw, Organic fooders who go so far as to eat only unfired, unground cereals that have been soaked in warm water (at less than 115 degrees or you'll kill the enzymes) for many hours to soften the seeds up and start them sprouting. This diet works and really helps a lot of people. Raw organic foodism is especially good for "holy joes," a sort of better-than-everyone-else person who enjoys great self-righteousness by owning this system. But raw fooding does not help all people nor solve all diseases because raw food irritates the digestive tracts of some people and in northern climates it is hard to maintain body heat on this diet because it is difficult to consume enough concentrated vegetable food in a raw state. And some raw fooders eat far too much fruit. I've seen them lose their teeth because of fruit's low mineral content, high sugar level and constant fruit acids in their mouths.

Then there are vegetarians of various varieties including vegans (vegetarians that will not eat dairy products and eggs), and then, there are their exact opposites, Atkins dieters focusing on protein and eating lots of meat. There's the Adelle Davis school, people eating whole grains, handfuls of vitamins, lots of dairy and brewer's yeast and wheat germ, and even raw liver. Then there's the Organic school. These folks will eat anything in any combination, just so long as it is organically produced, including organically raised beef, chicken, lamb, eggs, rabbit, wild meats, milk and dairy products, natural sea salt in large quantities and of course, organically grown fruits, vegetables grains and nuts. And what is "Organic?" The word means food raised in compliance with a set of rules contrived by a certification bureaucracy. When carefully analyzed, the somewhat illogical rules are not all that different in spirit than the rules of kashsruth or kosher. And the Organic certification bureaucrats aren't all that different than the rabbis who certify food as being kosher, either.

There are now millions of frightened Americans who, following the advice of mainstream Authority, have eliminated red meat from their diets and greatly reduced what they (mistakenly) understand as high-cholesterol foods.

All these diets work too—or some—and all demonstrate some of the truth.

The only area concerning health that contains more confusion and contradictory data than diet is vitamins. What a rats nest that is!

The Fundamental Principle

If you are a true believer in any of the above food religions, I expect that you will find my views unsettling. But what I consider "good diet" results from my clinical work with thousands of cases. It is what has worked with those cases. My eclectic views incorporate bits and pieces of all the above. In my own case, I started out by following the Organic school, and I was once a raw food vegetarian who ate nothing but raw food for six years. I also ate Macrobiotic for about one year until I became violently allergic to rice.

I have arrived at a point where I understand that each person's biochemistry is unique and each must work out their own diet to suit their life goals, life style, genetic predisposition and current state of health. There is no single, one, all-encompassing, correct diet. But, there is a single, basic, underlying Principle of Nutrition that is universally true. In its most simplified form, the basic equation of human health goes: Health = Nutrition / Calories. The equation falls far short of explaining the origin of each individuals diseases or how to cure diseases but Health = Nutrition / Calories does show the general path toward healthful eating and proper medicine.

All animals have the exact same dietary problem: finding enough nutrition to build and maintain their bodies within the limits of their digestive capacity. Rarely in nature (except for predatory carnivores) is there any significant restriction on the number of calories or serious limitation of the amount of low-nutrition foods available to eat. There's rarely any shortage of natural junk food on Earth. Except for domesticated house pets, animals are sensible enough to prefer the most nutritional fare available and tend to shun empty calories unless they are starving.

But humans are perverse, not sensible. Deciding on the basis of artificially-created flavors, preferring incipid textures, we seem to prefer junk food and become slaves to our food addictions. For example, in tropical countries there is a widely grown root crop, called in various places: tapioca, tavioca, manioc, or yuca. This interesting plant produces the greatest tonnage of edible, digestible, pleasant-tasting calories per acre compared to any other food crop I know. Manioc might seem the answer to human starvation because it will grow abundantly on tropical soils so infertile and/or so droughty that no other food crop will succeed there. Manioc will do this because it needs virtually nothing from the soil to construct itself with. And consequently, manioc puts next to nothing nourishing into its edible parts. The bland-tasting root is virtually pure starch, a simple carbohydrate not much different than pure corn starch. Plants construct starches from carbon dioxide gas obtained the air and hydrogen obtained from water. There is no shortage ever of carbon from CO_2 in the air and rarely a shortage of hydrogen from water. When the highly digestible starch in manioc is chewed, digestive enzymes readily convert it into sugar. Nutritionally there is virtually no difference between eating manioc and eating white sugar. Both are entirely empty calories.

If you made a scale from ideal to worst regarding the ratio of nutrition to calories, white sugar, manioc and most fats are at the extreme undesirable end. Frankly I don't know which single food might lie at the extreme positive end of the scale. Close to perfect might be certain leafy green vegetables that can be eaten raw. When they are grown on extremely fertile soil, some greens develop 20 or more percent completely digestible balanced protein with ideal ratios of all the essential amino acids, lots of vitamins, tons of minerals, all sorts of enzymes and other nutritional elements—and very few calories. You could continually fill your stomach to bursting with raw leafy greens and still have a hard time sustaining your body weight if that was all you ate. Maybe Popeye the Sailorman was right about eating spinach.

For the moment, lets ignore individual genetic inabilities to digest specific foods and also ignore the effects stress and enervation can have on our ability to extract nutrition out of the food we are eating. Without those factors to consider, it is correct to say that, to the extent one's diet contains the maximum potential amount of nutrition relative to the number of calories you are eating, to that extent a person will be healthy. To the extent the diet is degraded from that ideal, to that extent, disease will develop. Think about it!

Lessons *from* Nutritional Anthropology

The next logical pair of questions are: how healthy could good nutrition make people be, and, how much deviation from ideal nutrition could we allow ourselves before serious disease appears? Luckily, earlier in this century we could observe living answers to those questions (before the evidence disappeared). The answers are: we could be amazingly healthy, and, if we wish to enjoy excellent health we can afford to cut ourselves surprisingly little slack.

Prior to the Second World War there were several dozen sizable groups of extraordinarily healthy humans remaining on Earth. Today, their descendants are still in the same remote places, are speaking the same languages and possess more or less the same cultures. Only today they're watching satellite TV. wearing jeans, drinking colas— and their superior health has evaporated.

During the early part of this century, at the same era vitamins and other basic aspects of nutrition were being discovered, a few farsighted medical explorers sought out these hard-to-reach places with their legendarily healthy peoples to see what caused the legendary well-being they'd heard of. Enough evidence was collected and analyzed to derive some very valid principles.

First lets dismiss some apparently logical but incorrect explanations for the unusually good health of these isolated peoples. It wasn't racial, genetic superiority. There were extraordinarily healthy blacks, browns, Orientals, Amerinds, Caucasians. It wasn't living at high altitude; some lived at sea level. It wasn't temperate climates, some lived in the tropics, some in the tropics at sea level, a type of location generally thought to be quite unhealthful. It wasn't a small collection of genetically superior individuals, because when these peoples left their isolated locale and moved to the city, they rapidly began to lose their health. And it wasn't genetics because when a young couple from the isolated healthy village moved to town, their children born in town were as unhealthy as all the other kids.

And what do I mean by genuinely healthy? Well, imagine a remote village or a mountain valley or a far island settlement very difficult to get to, where there lived a thousand or perhaps ten thousand people. Rarely fewer, rarely more. Among that small population there were no medical doctors and no dentists, no drugs, no vaccinations, no antibiotics. Usually the isolation carried with it illiteracy and precluded contact with or awareness of modern science, so there was little or no notion of public hygiene. And this was before the era of antibiotics. Yet these unprotected, undoctored, unvaccinated peoples did not suffer and die from bacterial infections; and the women did not have to give birth to 13 children to get 2.4 to survive to breeding age—almost all the children made it through the gauntlet of childhood diseases. There was also virtually no degenerative disease like heart attacks, hardening of the arteries, senility, cancer, arthritis. There were few if any birth defects. In fact, there probably weren't any aspirin in the entire place. Oh, and there was very little mortality during childbirth, as little or less than we have today with all our hospitals. And the people uniformly had virtually perfect teeth and kept them all till death, but did not have toothbrushes nor any notion of dental hygiene. Nor did they have dentists or physicians. (Price, 1970)

And in those fortunate places the most common causes of death were accident (trauma) and old age. The typical life span was long into the 70s and in some places quite a bit longer. One fabled place, Hunza, was renowned for having an extraordinarily high percentage of vigorous and active people over 100 years old.

I hope I've made you curious. "How could this be?" you're asking. Well, here's why. First, everyone of those groups lived in places so entirely remote, so inaccessible that they were of necessity, virtually self-sufficient. They hardly traded at all with the outside world, and certainly they did not trade for bulky, hard-to-transport bulk foodstuffs. Virtually everything they ate was produced by themselves. If they were an agricultural people, naturally, everything they ate was natural: organic, whole, unsprayed and fertilized with whatever local materials seemed to produce enhanced plant growth. And, if they were agricultural, they lived on a soil body that possessed highly superior natural fertility. If not an agricultural people they lived by the sea and made a large portion of their diets sea foods. If their soil had not been extraordinarily fertile, these groups would not have enjoyed superior health and would have conformed to the currently widely-believed notion that before the modern era, people's lives were brutish, unhealthful, and short.

What is common between meat-eating Eskimos, isolated highland Swiss living on rye bread, milk and cheese; isolated Scottish island Celts with a dietary of oat porridge, kale and sea foods; highland central Africans (Malawi) eating sorghum, millet tropical root crops and all sorts of garden vegetables, plus a little meat and dairy; Fijians living on small islands in the humid tropics at sea level eating sea foods and garden vegetables. What they had in common was that their foods were all were at the extreme positive end of the Health = Nutrition / Calories scale. The agriculturists were on very fertile soil that grew extraordinarily nutrient-rich food, the sea food gatherers were obtaining their tucker from the place where all the fertility that ever was in the soil had washed out of the land had been transported—sea foods are also extraordinarily nutrient rich.

The group with the very best soil and consequently, the best health of all were, by lucky accident, the Hunza. I say "lucky" and "accident" because the Hunza and their resource base unknowingly developed an agricultural system that produced the most nutritious food that is possible to grow. The Hunza lived on what has been called super food. There are a lot of interesting books about the Hunza, some deserving of careful study. (Wrench, 1938; Rodale, 1949)

Finding Your Ideal Dietary

Anyone that is genuinely interested in having the best possible health should make their own study of the titles listed in the bibliography in the back of this book. After you do, award yourself a BS nutrition. I draw certain conclusions from this body of data. I think they help a person sort out the massive confusion that exists today about proper diet.

First principle: Homo Sapiens clearly can posses extreme health while eating very different dietary regimens. There is no one right diet for humans.

Before the industrial era almost everyone on Earth ate what was produced locally. Their dietary choices were pretty much restricted to those foods that were well adapted and productive in their region. Some places grew rye, others wheat, others millet, others rice. Some places supported cows, others goats, others had few on no domesticated animals. Some places produced a lot of fruits and vegetables. Others, did not. Whatever the local dietary, during thousands of years of eating that dietary natural selection prevailed; most babies that were allergic to or not able to thrive on the available dietary, died quickly. Probably of childhood bacterial infections. The result of this weeding out process was a population closely adapted to the available dietary of a particular locale.

This has interesting implications for Americans, most of whose ancestors immigrated from somewhere else; many of our ancestors also "hybridized" or crossed with immigrants from elsewhere. Trying to discover what dietary substances your particular genetic endowment is adapted to can be difficult and confusing. If both your parents were Italian and they were more or less pure Italian going way back, you might start out trying to eat wheat, olives, garlic, fava beans, grapes, figs, cow dairy. If pure German, try rye bread, cow dairy, apples, cabbage family vegetables. If Scottish, try oats, mutton, fish, sheep dairy and cabbage family vegetables. If Jewish, try goat dairy, wheat, olives and citrus. And certainly all the above ethnic derivations will thrive on many kinds of vegetables. Afro-Americans, especially dark-complexioned ones little mixed with Europeans, might do well to avoid wheat and instead, try sorghum, millet or tropical root crops like sweet potatoes, yams and taro.

Making it even more difficult for an individual to discover their optimum diet is the existence of genetic-based allergies and worse, developed allergies. Later in this chapter I will explain how a body can develop an allergy to a food that is probably irreversible. A weakened organ can also prevent digestion of a food or food group.

One more thing about adaptation to dietaries. Pre-industrial humans could only be extraordinarily healthy on the dietary they were adapted to if and only if that dietary also was extraordinarily high in nutrients. Few places on earth have naturally rich soil. Food grown on poor soil is poor in nutrition; that grown on rich soil is high in nutrition. People do not realize that the charts and tables in the backs of health books like Adelle Davis's Lets Cook It Right, are not really true. They are statistics. It is vital to keep in mind the old saying, "there are lies, there are damned lies, and then there are statistics. The best way to lie is with statistics."

Statistical tables of the nutrient content of foods were developed by averaging numerous samples of food from various soils and regions. These tables basically lie because they do not show the range of possibility between the different samples. A chart may state authoritatively that 100 grams of broccoli contains so many milligrams of calcium. What it does not say is that some broccoli samples contain only half that amount or even less, while other broccoli contains two or three times that amount. Since calcium is a vital nutrient hard to come by in digestible form, the high calcium broccoli is far better food than the low calcium sample. But both samples of broccoli appear and taste more or less alike. Both could even be organically grown. Yet one sample has a very positive ratio of nutrition to calories, the other is lousy food. (Schuphan, 1965) Here's another example I hope will really dent the certainties the Linda Clarkites. Potatoes can range in protein from eight to eleven percent, depending on the soil that produced them and if they were or were not irrigated. Grown dry (very low yielding) on semiarid soils, potatoes can be a high-protein staff of life. Heavily irrigated and fertilized so as to produce bulk yield instead of nutrition, they'll produce two or three times the tonnage, but at 8 percent protein instead of 11 percent. Not only does the protein content drop just as much as yield is boosted, the amino acid ratios change markedly, the content of scarce nutritional minerals drops massively, and the caloric content increases. In short, subsisting on irrigated commercially-grown potatoes, or on those grown on relatively infertile soils receiving abundant rainfall will make you fat and sick. They're a lot like manioc.

Here's another. Wheat can range from 7 to 19 percent protein. Before the industrial era ruined most wheat by turning it into white flour, wheat-eating peoples from regions where the cereal naturally contains abundant protein tended to be tall, healthy and long-lived. Wheat-eating humans from regions that produce low protein grain tended to be small, sickly and short-lived. (McCarrison, 1921, 1936, 1982; Albrecht, 1975)

Even cows have to pay attention to where their grass is coming from. Some green grass is over 15 percent protein and contains lots of calcium, phosphorus and magnesium to build strong bodies. Other equally or even better looking green grass contains only six or seven percent protein and contains little calcium, phosphorus or magnesium. Cows forced to eat only this poor type of grass can literally starve to death with full bellies. And they have a hard time breeding successfully. The reason for the difference: different soil fertility profiles. (Albrecht, 1975)

When people ate local, those living on fertile soils or getting a significant portion of their diet from the sea and who because of physical isolation from industrial foods did not make a practice of eating empty calories tended to live a long time and be very healthy. But those unfortunates on poor soils or with unwise cultural life-styles tended to be short-lived, diseased, small, weak, have bad teeth, and etc. The lesson here is that Homo Sapiens can adapt to many different dietaries, but like any other animal, the one thing we can't adapt to is a dietary deficient in nutrition.

So here's another "statistic" to reconsider. Most people believe that due to modern medical wonders, we live longer than we used to. Actually, that depends. Compared to badly nourished populations of a century ago, yes! We do. Chemical medicine keeps sickly, poorly nourished people going a lot longer (though one wonders about the quality of their dreary existences.) I hypothesize that before the time most farmers purchased and baked with white flour and sold their whole, unground wheat, many rural Americans (the ones on good soil, not all parts of North America have rich soil) eating from their own self-sufficient farms, lived as long or even longer than we do today. You also have to wonder who benefits from promulgating this mistaken belief about longevity. Who gets rich when we are sick? And what huge economic interests are getting rich helping make us sick?

The Human Comedy

I know most of my readers have been heavily indoctrinated about food and think they already know the truth about dietetics. I also know that so much information (and misinformation) is coming out about diet that most of my readers are massively confused about the subject. These are two powerful reasons many readers will look with disbelief at what this chapter has to say and take no action on my data, even to prove me wrong.

Let me warn you. There is a deep-seated human tendency to put off taking responsibilities, beautifully demonstrated by this old joke.

A 14 year old boy was discovered masturbating by his father, who said, "son, you shouldn't do that! If you keep it up you'll eventually go blind!"

"But father," came the boy's quick reply. "It feels good. How about if I don't quit until I need to wear glasses?"

The Organic Versus Chemical Feud

Now, regrettably, and at great personal risk to my reputation, I must try to puncture the very favorite belief of food religionists, the doctrine that organically grown food is as nutritious as food can possibly be, Like Woody Allen's brown-rice-eating friends, people think if you eat Organic foods, you will inevitably live a very long time and be very healthy. Actually, the Organic vs. chemical feud is in many ways false. Many (not all) samples of organically grown food are as low or lower in nutrition as foods raised with chemical fertilizers. Conversely, wisely using chemical fertilizers (not pesticides) can greatly increase the nutritional value of food. Judiciously used Organic fertilizing substances can also do that as well or better. And in either case, using chemical fertilizers or so-called organic fertilizers, to maximize nutrition the humus content of the soil must be maintained. But, raising soil organic matter levels too high can result in a massive reduction in the nutritional content of the food being grown–a very frequent mistake on the part of Organic devotees. In other words, growing nutrition is a science, and is not a matter of religion.

The food I fed to my daughter in childhood, though Organic according to Rodale and the certification bureaucrats, though providing this organic food to my family and clients gave me a feeling of self-righteousness, was not grown with an understanding of the nutritional consequences of electing to use one particular Organic fertilizing substance over another. So we and a lot of regional Organic market gardeners near us that we bought from, were raising food that was far from ideally nutritious. At least though, our food was free of pesticide residues.

The real dichotomy in food is not "chemical" fertilizer versus "Organic," It is between industrial food and quality food. What I mean by industrial food is that which is raised with the intention of maximizing profit or yield. There is no contradiction between raising food that the "rabbis" running Organic certification bureaucracies would deem perfectly "kosher" and raising that same food to make the most possible money or the biggest harvest. When a farmer grows for money, they want to produce the largest number of bushels, crates, tons, bales per acre. Their criteria for success is primarily unit volume. Many gardeners think the same way. To maximize bulk yield they build soil fertility in a certain direction (organically or chemically) and choose varieties that produce greater bulk. However, nature is ironic in this respect. The most nutritious food is always lower yielding. The very soil management practices that maximize production simultaneously reduce nutrition.

The real problem we are having about our health is not that there are residues of pesticides in our food. The real problem is that there are only residues of nutrition left in our foods. Until our culture comes to understand this and realizes that the health costs of accepting less than optimum food far exceeds the profits made by growing bulk, it will not be possible to frequently find the ultimate of food quality in the marketplace, organically grown or not. It will not be possible to find food that is labeled or identified according to its real nutritional value. The best I can say about Organic food these days is that it probably is no less nutritious than chemically-grown food while at least it is free of pesticide residues.

The Poor Start

For this reason it makes sense to take vitamins and food supplements, to be discussed in the next chapter. And because our food supply, Organic or "conventional," is far from optimum, if a person wants to be and remain healthy and have a life span that approaches their genetic potential (and that potential, it seems, approaches or exceeds a century), it is essential that empty calories are rigorously avoided.

An accurate and quick-to-respond indicator of how well we are doing in terms of getting enough nutrition is the state of our teeth. One famous dentally-oriented nutritional doctor, Melvin Page, suggested that as long as overall nutrition was at least 75 percent of perfection, the body chemistry could support healthy teeth and gums until death. By healthy here Page means free of cavities, no bone loss around the teeth (no wobblers), no long-in-the-teeth mouths from receding gums, no gum diseases at all. But when empty calories or devitalized foods or misdigestion cuts our nutrient intake we begin experiencing tooth decay, gum disease and bone loss in the jaw. How are your teeth?

I suppose you could say that I have a food religion, but mine is to eat so that the equation Nutrition = Health / Calories is strongly in my favor.

Back to my daughter's teeth. Yes, I innocently fed her less than ideally nutritious food, but at that time I couldn't buy ideal food even had I known what I wanted, nor did I have any scientific idea of how to produce ideal food, nor actually, could I have done so on the impoverished, leached-out clay soil at Great Oaks School even had I known how. The Organic doctrine says that you can build a Garden of 'Eatin with large quantities of compost until any old clay pit or gravel heap produces highly nutritious food. This idea is not really true. Sadly, what is true about organic matter in soil is that when it is increased very much above the natural level one finds in untilled soil in the climate you're working with, the nutritional content of the food begins to drop markedly. I know this assertion is shocking and perhaps threatening to those who believe in the Organic system; I am sorry.

But there is another reason my daughter's teeth were not perfect, probably could not have been perfect no matter what we fed her, and why she will probably have at least some health problems as she ages no matter how perfectly she may choose to eat from here on. My daughters had what Dr. G.T. Wrench called "a poor start." Not as poor as it could have been by any means, but certainly less than ideal.

You see, the father has very little to do with the health of the child, unless he happens to carry some particularly undesirable gene. It is the mother who has the job of constructing the fetus out of prepartum nourishment and her own body's nutritional reserves. The female body knows from trillenia of instinctual experience that adequate nutrition from the current food supply during pregnancy cannot always be assured, so the female body stores up very large quantities of minerals and vitamins and enzymes against that very possibility. When forming a fetus these reserves are drawn down and depleted. It is virtually impossible during the pregnancy itself for a mother to extract sufficient nutrition from current food to build a totally healthy fetus, no matter how nourishing the food she is eating may be. Thus a mother-to-be needs to be spending her entire childhood and her adolescence (and have adequate time between babies), building and rebuilding her reserves.

A mother-to-be also started out at her own birth with a vitally important stock of nutritional reserves, reserves put there during her own fetal development. If that "start" was less than ideal, the mother-to-be (as fetus) got "pinched" and nutritionally shortchanged in certain, predictable ways. Even minor mineral fetal deficiencies degrade the bone structure: the fetus knows it needs nutritional reserves more than it needs to have a full-sized jaw bone or a wide pelvic girdle, and when deprived of maximum fetal nourishment, these non-vital bones become somewhat smaller. Permanently. If mineral deficiencies continue into infancy and childhood, these same bones continue to be shortchanged, and the child ends up with a very narrow face, a jaw bone far too small to hold all the teeth, and in women, a small oven that may have trouble baking babies. More importantly, those nutrient reserves earmarked especially for making babies are also deficient. So a deficient mother not only shows certain structural evidence of physiological degeneration, but she makes deficient babies. A deficient female baby at birth is unlikely to completely overcome her bad start before she herself has children.

So with females, the quality of a whole lifetime's nutrition, and the life-nutrition of her mother (and of her mother's mother as well) has a great deal to do with the outcome of a pregnancy. The sins of the mother can really be visited unto the third and fourth generation.

This reality was powerfully demonstrated in the 1920s by a medical doctor, Francis Pottenger. He was not gifted with a good bedside manner. Rather than struggling with an unsuccessful clinical practice, Dr. Pottenger decided to make his living running a medical testing laboratory in Pasadena, California. Dr. Pottenger earned his daily bread performing a rather simple task, assaying the potency of adrenal hormone extracts. At that time, adrenaline, a useful drug to temporarily rescue people close to death, was extracted from the adrenal glands of animals. However, the potency of these crude extracts varied greatly. Being a very powerful drug, it was essential to measure exactly how strong your extract was so its dosage could be controlled.

Quantitative organic chemistry was rather crude in those days. Instead of assaying in a test tube, Dr. Pottenger kept several big cages full of cats that he had adrenalectomized. Without their own adrenals, the cats could not live more than a short time by finding out how much extract was required to keep the cats from failing, he could measure the strength of the particular batch.

Dr. Pottenger's cats were economically valuable so he made every effort to keep them healthy, something that proved to be disappointingly difficult. He kept his cats clean, in airy, bright quarters, fed them to the very best of his ability on pasteurized whole milk, slaughterhouse meat and organs (cats in the wild eat organ meats first and there are valuable vitamins and other substances in organ meats that don't exist in muscle tissue). The meat was carefully cooked to eliminate any parasites, and the diet was supplemented with cod liver oil. However, try as he might, Pottenger's cats were sickly, lived short and had to be frequently replaced. Usually they bred poorly and died young of bacterial infections, there being no antibiotics in the 1920s. I imagine Dr. Pottenger was constantly visiting the animal shelter and perhaps even paid quarters out the back door to a steady stream of young boys who brought him cats in burlap sacks from who knows where, no questions asked.

Dr. Pottenger's assays must have been accurate, for his business grew and grew. Eventually he needed more cats than he had cages to house, so he built a big, roofed, on-the-ground pen outdoors. Because he was overworked, he was less careful about the feeding of these extra animals. They got the same pasteurized milk and cod-liver oil, but he did not bother to cook their slaughterhouse meat. Then, a small miracle happened. This poorly cared for cage of cats fed on uncooked meat became much healthier than the others, suffering far fewer bacterial infections or other health problems. Then another miracle happened. Dr. Pottenger began to meditate on the first miracle.

It occurred to him that cats in the wild did not cook their food; perhaps cats had a digestive system that couldn't process or assimilate much out of cooked food. Perhaps the problem he had been having was not because the cats were without adrenal glands but because they were without sustenance, suffering a sort of slow starvation in the midst of plenty. So Dr. Pottenger set up some cat feeding experiments.

There were four possible combinations of his regimen: raw meat and unpasteurized milk; raw meat and pasteurized milk; cooked meat and raw milk; cooked meat and pasteurized milk, this last one being what he had been feeding all along. So he divided his cats into four groups and fed each group differently. The first results of Pottenger's experiments were revealed quickly though the most valuable results took longer to see. The cats on raw meat and raw milk did best. The ones on raw meat and pasteurized milk did okay but not as well. The ones on cooked meat and raw milk did even less well and those on all cooked food continued to do as poorly as ever.

Clearly, cats can't digest cooked food; all animals do better fed on what they can digest. A lot of people have taken Pottenger's data and mistakenly concluded that humans also should eat only raw food. This idea is debatable. However, the most important result of the cat experiments took years to reveal itself and is not paid much attention to, probably because its implications are very depressing. Dr. Pottenger continued his experiments for several generations. It was the transgenerational changes that showed the most valuable lesson. Over several generations, the cats on all raw foods began to alter their appearance. Their faces got wider, their pelvic girdles broader, bones solider, teeth better. They began to breed very successfully.

After quite a few generations, the healthiest group, the one on all raw foods, seemed to have improved as much as it could. So Dr. Pottenger took some of these cats and began feeding them only cooked food to study the process of nutritional degeneration. After three "de"generations on cooked fodder the group had deteriorated so much that the animals could barely breed. Their faces had become narrow, their teeth crooked, their pelvic girdles narrow, their bones and body structure very small, and their dispositions poor. Mothers wouldn't nurse their young and sometimes became cannibalistic. They no longer lived very long.

Before the degenerating group completely lost the ability to breed, Pottenger began to again feed them all raw food. It took four generations on a perfect, raw food diet before some perfect appearing individuals showed up in the group. It takes longer to repair the damage than it does to cause it and it takes generations of unflagging persistence.

I think much the same process has happened to humans in this century. With the invention of the roller mill and the consequent degradation of our daily bread to white flour; with the birth of industrial farming and the generalized lowering of the nutritional content of all of our crops; our overall ratio of nutrition to calories worsened. Then it worsened again because we began to have industrial food manufacturing and national brand prepared food marketing systems; we began subsisting on devitalized, processed foods. The result has been an even greater worsening of our ratio of nutrition to calories.

And just like Pottenger's cats, we civilized humans in so-called advanced countries are losing the ability to breed, our willingness (or the energy) to mother our young; we're losing our good humor in the same way Pottenger's degenerated cats became bad tempered. As a group we feel so poorly that we desperately need to feel better fast, and what better way to do that than with drugs. Is it any wonder that the United States, the country furthest down the road of industrial food degeneration, spends 14 percent of its gross domestic product on medical services. Any wonder that so many babies are born by Cesarean, any wonder that so many of our children have crooked teeth needing an orthodontist? The most depressing aspect of this comes into view when considering that Pottenger's cats took four generations on perfect food to repair most of the nutritional damage.

In the specific case of my daughter, I know some things about the nutritional history of her maternal ancestors. My daughter's grandmother grew up on a Saskatchewan farm. Though they certainly grew their own rich wheat on virgin semi-arid prairie soil, I'm sure the family bought white flour at the store for daily use. Still, there was a garden and a cow producing raw milk and free-range fertile eggs and chicken and other animals. There probably were lots of canned vegetables in winter, canned but still highly nutritious because of the fertility of their prairie garden. My mother consequently had perfect teeth until the Great Depression forced her to live for too many years on lard and white bread.

During this time of severe malnutrition she had her three babies. The first one got the best of her nutritional reserves. The second, born after the worst of the malnutrition, was very small and weak and had a hard time growing up. Fortunately for me, for a few years before I (the last child) was born, the worst of the economic times had past and the family had been living on a farm. There were vegetables and fresh raw milk and fruit. My mother had two good years to rebuild her nutritional reserves. But "Grannybell" did not manage to replace enough. Shortly after I was born my mother lost every one of her teeth all at once. The bone just disappeared around them.

Thus, I was born deficient. And my childhood and adolescent nutrition was poor too: soda crackers, pasteurized processed artificial cheese, evaporated milk from cans, hotdogs and canned beans, hotdogs and cabbage. It wasn't until I was pregnant with my first baby that I started to straighten up my diet. I continued eating very well after my first daughter, so my youngest daughter had another three years of good diet to draw on. Thus both my own daughters got a somewhat better start than I had had.

My teeth were not as good as my mother's had been before those years of malnutrition took them all. Instead of perfect straight undecayed teeth like a healthy farm girl should have, mine were somewhat crowded, with numerous cavities. My jaw bone had not received enough minerals to develop to its full size. My pelvic girdle also was smaller than my mother's was. I had had a poor start.

My daughters did better. The older one (the first child typically gets the best of the nutritional reserves) has such a wide jaw that there are small spaces between her teeth. My second daughter has only one crooked tooth, she has wider, more solid hips, stronger bones and a broader face than I do. If my younger daughter will but from this point in her life, eat perfectly and choose her food wisely to responsibly avoid empty calories and maximize her ratio of nutrition to calories, her daughter (if she gives us granddaughters as her older sister already has done) may exhibit the perfect physiology that her genes carry.

Along the lines of helping you avoid empty calories I will give you some information about various common foods that most people don't know and that most books about food and health don't tell, or misunderstand.

Butter, Margarine & Fats *in* General

Recently, enormous propaganda has been generated against eating butter. It's been smeared in the health magazines as a saturated animal fat, one containing that evil substance, cholesterol. Many people are now avoiding it and instead, using margarine.

Composition of Oils			
	Saturated	Monosaturated	Unsaturated
Butter	66%	30%	4%
Coconut Oil	87%	6%	2%
Cottonseed Oil	26%	18%	52%
Olive Oil	13%	74%	8%
Palm Oil	49%	37%	9%
Soybean Oil	14%	24%	58%
Sunflower Oil	4%	8%	83%
Safflower Oil	3%	5%	87%
Sesame Oil	5%	9%	80%
Peanut Oil	6%	12%	76%
Corn Oil	3%	7%	84%

This is a major and serious misunderstanding. First of all, margarine is almost indigestible, chemically very much like shortening–an artificially saturated or hydrogenated vegetable fat. Hydrogenated fats can't be properly broken down by the body's digestive enzymes, adding to the body's toxic load. Margarine, being a chemically-treated vegetable oil with artificial yellow color and artificial flavorings to make it seem like butter, also releases free radicals in the body that accelerate aging. So, to avoid the dangers of eating cholesterol-containing butter, people eat something far worse for them!

There are severe inconsistencies with the entire "cholesterol-is-evil" theory. Ethnic groups like the Danes, who eat enormous quantities of cholesterol-containing foods, have little circulatory disease. Actually, the liver itself produces cholesterol; its presence in the blood is an important part of the body chemistry. Cholesterol only becomes a problem because of deranged body chemistry due to the kind of overall malnutrition Americans usually experience on their junk food diets. Avoiding cholesterol in foods does little good, but eating a low-fat, low-sugar, complex-carbohydrate (whole foods) diet high in minerals does lower blood cholesterol enormously.

Actually, high quality fresh (not rancid) butter in moderate quantities is about the finest fat a person could eat. But high quality butter is almost unobtainable. First of all, it has to be raw, made from unpasteurized cream. Second, butter can contain very high levels of fat-soluble vitamins, but doesn't have to. Vitamin-rich butter's color is naturally bright yellow, almost orange. This color does not come from a test tube. Pale yellow butter as is found in the commercial trade was probably almost white before it was artificially tinted. Butter from grass-pastured cows naturally changes from yellow-orange to white and back again through the year as the seasons change. Spring grass, growing in the most intense sunlight of the year contains very high levels of chlorophyll and vitamins. Cows eating this grass put high levels of vitamins A and D into their cream, evidenced by the orange color of vitamin A. By July, natural butter has degraded to medium-yellow in color. By August, it is pale yellow. Industrial dairy cows fed exclusively on hay or artificial, processed feeds (lacking in these vitamins), produce butterfat that is almost white.

I prefer to obtain my butter from a neighbor who has several dairy cows grazing on fertile bottom land pasture. We always freeze a year's supply in late spring when butter is at its best. Interestingly, that is also the time of year when my neighbor gets the most production from her cows and is most willing to part with 25 pounds of extra butter.

In general, fats are poor foods that should be avoided. Their ratio of nutrition to calories is absolutely the worst of all food types, except perhaps for pure white sugar, which is all calories and absolutely no nutrition (this is also true for other forms of sugar. Honey, too, contains almost no nutrition.). Gram for gram, fats contain many more calories than do sugars or starches. Yet gram for gram, fats contain virtually no nutrition except for small quantities of essential fatty acids.

The perverse reason people like to eat fats is that they are very hard to digest and greatly slow the digestive action of the stomach. Another way of saying that is that they have a very high satiety value. Fats make a person feel full for a long time because their presence in the stomach makes it churn and churn and churn. Fats coat proteins and starches and delay their digestion, often causing them to begin fermenting (starches) or putrefying (proteins) in the digestive tract.

The best fats contain high levels of monosaturated vegetable oils that have never been exposed to heat or chemicals—like virgin olive oil. Use small quantities of olive oil for salad dressing. Monosaturated fats also have far less tendency to go rancid than any other type. Vegetable oils with high proportions of unsaturated fats, the kind that all the authorities push because they contain no cholesterol, go rancid rapidly upon very brief exposure to air. The danger here is that rancidity in vegetable oil is virtually unnoticeable. Rancid animal fat on the other hand, smells "off." Eating rancid oil is a sure-fire way to accelerate aging, invite degenerative conditions in general, and enhance the likelihood of cancer. I recommend that you use only high-quality virgin olive oil, the only generally-available fat that is largely monosaturated. (Pearson and Shaw, 1983)

When you buy vegetable oil, even olive oil, get small bottles so you use them up before the oil has much time being exposed to air (as you use the oil air fills the bottle) or, if you buy olive oil in a large can to save money, immediately upon opening it, transfer the oil to pint jars filled to the very brim to exclude virtually all air, and seal the jars securely. In either case, keep now-opened, in-use small bottles of oil in the refrigerator because rancidity is simply the combination of oil with oxygen from the air and this chemical reaction is accelerated at warmer temperatures and slowed greatly at cold ones.

Chemical reactions typically double in speed with every 10 degrees C. increase in temperature. So oil goes rancid about six times faster at normal room temperature than it does in the fridge. If you'll think about the implications of this data you'll see there are two powerful reasons not to fry food. One, the food is coated with oil and gains in satiety value at the expense of becoming relatively indigestible and productive of toxemia. Secondly, if frying occurs at 150 degrees Centigrade and normal room temperature is 20 degrees Centigrade, then oil goes rancid 2 to the 13th power faster in the frying pan, or about 8,200 times faster. Heating oil for only ten minutes in a hot skillet induces as much rancidity as about 6 weeks of sitting open and exposed to air at room temperature. Think about that the next time you're tempted to eat something from a fast food restaurant where the hot fat in the deep fryer has been reacting with oxygen all day, or even for several days.

Back to butter, where we started. If you must have something traditionally northern European on your bread, you are far better off to use butter, not margarine. However, Mediterranean peoples traditionally dip their bread in high-quality extra-virgin olive oil that smells and tastes like olives. It's delicious, why not try it. But best yet, put low-sugar fruit preserves on your toast or develop a taste for dry toast. Probably the finest use for butter is melted over steamed vegetables. This way only small quantities are needed and the fat goes on something that is otherwise very easy to digest so its presence will not produce as many toxins in the digestive tract.

Milk, Meat, & Other Protein Foods

Speaking of butter, how about milk? The dairy lobby is very powerful in North America. Its political clout and campaign contributions have the governments of both the United States and especially that of Canada eating out of its hand (literally), providing the dairy industry with price supports. Because of these price supports, in Canada cheese costs half again more than it does in the United States. The dairy lobby is also very cozy with the medical profession so licensed nutritionists constantly bombard us with "drink milk" and "cheese is good for you" propaganda.

And people naturally like dairy foods. They taste good and are fat-rich with a high satiety value. Dairy makes you feel full for a long time. Dairy is also high in protein; protein is hard to digest and this too keeps one feeling full for a long time. But many people, especially those from cultures who traditionally (genetically) didn't have dairy cows, particularly Africans, Asians and Jews, just do not produce the enzymes necessary to digest cow's milk. Some individuals belonging to these groups can digest goats milk. Some can't digest any kind except human breast milk. And some can digest fermented milk products like yogurt and kiefer. Whenever one eats a protein food that is not fully digestible, it putrefies in the digestive tract, with all the bad consequences previously described.

But no one, absolutely no one can fully digest pasteurized cow's milk, which is what most people use because they have been made to fear cow-transmitted diseases and/or they are forced to use pasteurized dairy products by health authorities. I suspect drinking pasteurized milk or eating cheese made from pasteurized milk is one of the reasons so many people develop allergic reactions to milk. Yet many states do not allow unpasteurized dairy to be sold, even privately between neighbors. To explain all this, I first have to explain a bit more about protein digestion in general and then talk about allergies and how they can be created.

Proteins are long, complex molecules, intricate chains whose individual links are amino acids. Proteins are the very stuff of life. All living protoplasm, animal or plant, is largely composed of proteins. There are virtually an infinite number of different proteins but all are composed of the same few dozen amino acids hooked together in highly variable patterns. Amino acids themselves are highly complex organic molecules too. The human body custom-assembles all its proteins from amino acids derived from digesting protein foods, and can also manufacture small quantities of certain of its own amino acids to order, but there are eight amino acids it cannot make and these are for that reason called essential amino acids. Essential amino acids must be contained in the food we eat. .

Few proteins are water soluble. When we eat proteins the digestive apparatus must first break them down into their water-soluble components, amino acids, so these can pass into the blood and then be reassembled into the various proteins the body uses. The body has an interesting mechanism to digest proteins; it uses enzymes. An enzyme is like the key for a lock. It is a complex molecule that latches to a protein molecule and then breaks it apart into amino acids. Then the enzyme finds yet another protein molecule to free. Enzymes are efficient, reusable many many times.

Enzymes that digest proteins are effective only in the very acid environment of the stomach, are manufactured by the pancreas and are released when protein foods are present. The stomach then releases hydrochloric acid and churns away like a washing machine, mixing the enzymes and the acid with the proteins until everything has digested.

So far so good. That's how it's supposed to be. But Dr. Henry Bieler, who wrote Food Is Your Best Medicine, came up with the finest metaphor I know of to explain how protein digestion goes wrong. He compared all proteins to the white of an egg (which is actually a form of protein). When raw and liquid, the long chains of albumen (egg white) proteins are in their natural form. However, cook the egg and the egg white both solidifies and becomes smaller. What has happened is that the protein chains have shriveled and literally tied themselves into knots. Once this happens, pancreatic enzymes no longer fit and cannot separate all the amino acids. Cooked proteins may churn and churn and churn in the presence of acid and pancreatic enzymes but they will not digest completely. Part becomes water soluble; part does not.

But, indigestible protein is still subject to an undesirable form of consumption in the gut. Various bacteria make their home in our airless, warm intestines. Some of these live on protein. In the process of consuming undigested proteins, they release highly toxic substances. They poison us.

What is true of the white of an egg is also true of flesh foods and dairy. Raw meat and raw fish are actually easily digestible foods and if not wrongly combined will not produce toxemia in a person that still has a strong pancreas. However, eating raw meat and fish can be a dicey proposition, both for reasons of cultural sensibility (people think it is disgusting) and because there may be living parasites in uncooked flesh that can attack, sicken and even kill people. It has been argued that a healthy stomach containing its proper degree of acidity provides an impenetrable barrier to parasites. Perhaps. But how many of us are that healthy these days? Cooked flesh and fish seems more delicious to our refined, civilized sensibilities, but are a poor food.

In my household we have no moral objection to eating meat. We do have an ethical objection in that meat eating does not contribute to our health. But still, we do eat it. A few times a year, for traditional celebrations we may invite the children over and cook a turkey. A few times for Thanksgiving when the children were going through their holier-than-thou vegetarian stage, I purchased the largest, thickest porterhouse steak I could find at the natural meat store and ate it medium-rare, with relish. It was delicious. It made me feel full for hours and hours and hours. I stayed flat on the couch and groggily worked on digesting it all evening. After that I'd had enough of meat to last for six months.

When milk is pasteurized, the proteins in it are also altered in structure. Not so severely as egg white is altered by cooking because pasteurization happens at a lower temperature. But altered none the less. And made less digestible. Pasteurizing also makes milk calcium far less assimilable. That's ironic because so many people are drinking milk because they fear they need more calcium to avoid osteoporosis and to give their children good teeth. What pasteurized milk actually does to their children is make them calcium deficient and makes the children toxic, provoking many colds, ear infections, sinusitis, inflammations of the tonsils and lung infections, and, induces an allergy to milk in the children.

The Development *of* Allergies

There are three ways a body can become allergic. (1) It can have a genetic predisposition for a specific allergy to start with. (2) It can be repeatedly exposed to an irritating substance such as pollen when, at the same time, the body's mechanism for dealing with irritations is weakened. Generally weak adrenals causes this because the adrenal's job is to produce hormones that reduce inflammation. Once the irritating substance succeeds at producing a significant inflammation, a secondary reaction may be set up, called an allergy. Once established, an allergy is very hard to get rid of. (3) In a way very similar to the second, but instead of being irritated by an external substance, it is irritated by repeatedly failing to properly, fully digest something. Pasteurized milk for example, basically impossible to completely digest even in its low-fat form, often sets up an allergy that applies to other forms of cow's milk, even raw, unpasteurized cow's milk or yogurt. Eating too much white flour can eventually set off a wheat allergy. My husband developed a severe allergy to barley after drinking too much home-brewed beer; he also became highly intolerant to alcohol. Now he has allergic reactions to both alcohol and barley. And gets far sicker from drinking beer (two separate allergies) than from wheat beer, hard liquor or wine (only one allergy).

Eating too much of any single food, or repeatedly eating too much of an otherwise very good food at one time, can eventually overwhelm the body's ability to digest it fully. Then, the finest whole food products may set up an allergic reaction. Worse, this allergic reaction itself subsequently prevents proper digestion even when only moderate quantities are eaten.

An allergy may not be recognized as an allergy because it may not manifest as the instant skin rash or stuffy nose or swollen glands or sticky eyes. that people usually think of when they think "allergic reaction." Food allergies can cause many kinds of symptoms, from sinusitis to psychosis, from asthma to arthritis, from hyperactivity to depression, insomnia to narcolepsy–and commonly the symptoms don't manifest immediately after eating. Frequently, allergic reactions are so low grade as to be unnoticeable and may not produce an observable condition until many years of their grinding down the vital force has passed. When the condition finally appears it is hard to associate it with some food that has been consumed for years, apparently with impunity.

Thus it is that many North Americans have developed allergies to wheat, dairy, soy products (because many soy foods are very hard to digest), corn and eggs. These are such common, widespread, frequently found allergies that anyone considering a dietary cause of their complaints might just cut all these foods out of the diet for a few weeks just to see what happens. And individuals may be allergic to anything from broccoli to bacon, strawberries to bean sprouts. Unraveling food allergies sometimes requires the deductions of a Sherlock Holmes.

However, food allergies are very easy to cure if you can get the suffered to take the medicine. Inevitably, allergic reactions vanish in about five days of abstinence. Anyone with sufficient self-discipline to water fast for five days can cure themselves of all food allergies at one step. Then, by a controlled, gradual reintroduction of foods, they can discover which individual items cause trouble. See Coca's Pulse Test in the Appendix where you'll find step-by-step instructions for allergy testing that are less rigorous, not requiring a preliminary fast.

Flour, & Other Matters Relating To Seeds

One of the largest degradations to human health was caused by the roller mill. This apparently profitable machine permitted the miller to efficiently separate wheat flour into three components: bran, germ and endosperm. Since bread made without bran and germ is lighter and appears more "upper class" it became instantly popular. Flour without germ and bran also had an industrial application–it could be stored virtually forever without being infested by insects because white flour does not contain enough nutrition to support life. Most health conscious people are aware that white flour products won't support healthful human life either.

Essentially, white flour's effect on humans is another demonstration of Health = Nutrition / Calories. When the bran and germ are discarded, remaining are the calories and much of the protein, lacking are many vitamins and minerals and other vital nutritional substances.

Whole wheat bread has been called the staff of life. In ages past, healthy cultures have made bread the predominant staple in their diet. Does that mean you can just go to the bakery and buy whole grain bread, or go to the health food store and buy organically grown whole wheat flour, bake your own, and be as healthy as the ancients? Sorry, the answer is almost certainly no. There are pitfalls, many of them, waiting for the unwary.

White flour has one other advantage over whole wheat flour. It not only remains free of insect infestation, it doesn't become stale (meaning rancid). In the wheat germ (where the embryo resides) there is considerable oil, containing among other things, about the best natural source of vitamin E. This oil is highly unsaturated and once the seed is ground the oil goes rancid in a matter of days. Whole wheat flour kept on the unrefrigerated shelf of the store is almost certainly rancid. A lot of its other vitamin content has been oxidized too. If the wheat flour had flowed directly from the grinder into an airtight sack and from there directly to the freezer, if it had been flash frozen and kept extremely cold, it might have a storage life of some months. Of course that was not the case. Maybe you're lucky and your health food store is one of the very few that has its own small-scale flour mill and grinds daily. Probably not.

How about your baker's whole wheat bread? Where does the baker get flour? From the wholesaler's or distributor's warehouse! In fifty pound kraftpaper sacks! How much time had elapsed from milling to wholesaler to baker to baking? The answer has to be in the order of magnitude of weeks. And it might be months. Was the flour stored frozen? Or airtight? Of course not.

If you want bread made from freshly ground flour you are almost certainly have to grind and bake it yourself. Is it worth the trouble? You bet. Once you've tasted real bread you'll instantly see by comparison what stale, rancid whole wheat flour tastes like. Freshly ground flour makes bread that can be the staff of life and can enormously upgrade your health–if the wheat you use is any good.

But before we talk about wheat quality, a more few words of warning. If you think wheat goes rancid rapidly, rye is even worse. Rye flour goes bad so fast that when you buy it in the store it usually is the rye equivalent of white wheat flour. The germ has been removed. The bag may not say so. But it probably has. If you are going to make rye breads, even more reason to grind your own. Corn meal from the grocery store has usually been degerminated too. If it hasn't been, the oil in the seed's germ has probably gone rancid.

Grinding flour at home is easy these days. There is an abundance of at-home milling products and no shortage of hype about them. You'll find staunch advocates of stone mills. These produce the finest-textured flour, but are costly. The sales pitch is that stones grind at low temperature and do not damage the oils (remember the development of rancidity is a function of temperature) or the vitamins, which are also destroyed at high temperature. This assertion is half true. If you are going to store your flour it is far better to grind it cool. However, if you are, as we do, going to immediately bake your flour, what difference does it make if it gets a little warm before baking. That only accelerates the action of the yeast.

On the negative side, stone mills grind slowly and are very fussy about which grains they will grind. If the cereal is a bit moist or if the seed being ground is a little bit oily, the mill becomes instantly blocked.

Steel burr mills grind fast and coarsely and are inexpensive. Coarse flour makes heavy bread. The metal grinding faces tend to wear out and have to be replaced occasionally–if they can be replaced. Breads on the heavy side are still delicious; for many years I made bread with an inexpensive steel burr mill attachment that came with my juicer.

Some steel burr mills will also grind oily seed like sesame and sunflower. However, oily seeds can be ground far more easily half-a-cup at a time in a little inexpensive electric spice/coffee mill, the sort with a single fast-spinning propeller.

I currently think the best compromise are hammermills. The grain dribbles into a chamber full of fast-spinning teeth that literally pound the grain into powder. Since air flows through with the grain the flour is not heated very much. This type of mill is small, very fast, intermediate in price between steel mills and stone mill, lasts a long time, but when grinding, sounds like a Boeing 747 about to take off. It is essential to wear hearing protectors when using it.

Awareness of bread quality is growing. One excellent new U.S. business, called Great Harvest Bakery is a fast-growing national franchise chain. They bake and sell only whole grain breads; all their wheat flour is freshly ground daily on the premises in the back. Unfortunately, as of the writing of this book, they do not grind their rye flour but bring it in sacks. I can't recommend their rye breads. The founder of Great Harvest is a knowledgeable buyer who fully understands my next topic, which is that wheat is not wheat.

There are great differences between hard bread wheats; being organically grown is no cure all for making good or nutritious bread. Great Harvest understands this and uses top quality grain that is also Organic.

When I first started making my own bread from my own at-home-ground flour I was puzzled by variations in the dough. Sometimes the bread rose well and was spongy after baking like I wanted it to be. Sometimes it kneaded stickily and ended up flat and crumbly like a cake. Since I had done everything the same way except that I may have bought my wheat berries from different health food stores, I began to investigate the subject of wheat quality.

The element in the cereal that forms the rubbery sponge in risen bread so it doesn't crumble and rises high without collapsing, is gluten. The word glue derives from gluten. The gluten content of various wheats varies. Bread bakers use "hard wheat" because of its high gluten content. Gluten is a protein and gluten comprises most of the protein in bread wheat; the protein content and the gluten content are almost identical.

Try this. Ask your health food store buyer or owner what the protein content is of the hard red wheat seeds they're selling. You'll almost certainly get a puzzled look and your answer will almost certainly be, "we have Organic and conventional." Demand that the store buyer ask this question of their distributor/wholesaler and then report back to you. If the distributor deigns to answer, the answer will be the same–I sell Organic or conventional hard red wheat. Period. When I got these non-answers I looked further and discovered that hard bread wheats run from about 12 percent protein to about 19 percent and this difference has everything to do with the soil fertility (and to an extent the amount of rainfall during the season), and almost nothing to do with Organic or conventional.

This difference also has everything to do with how your dough behaves and how your bread comes out. And how well your bread nourishes you. Thirteen percent wheat will not make a decent loaf–fourteen percent is generally considered #2 quality and comprises the bulk of cheap bread grain. When you hear in the financial news that a bushel of wheat is selling for a certain price, they mean #2. Bakers compete for higher protein lots and pay far higher prices for more protein.

We prefer our bread about 25% rye, but rye contains no gluten at all. Mix any rye flour into fourteen percent wheat flour and the dough becomes very heavy, won't rise, and after baking, crumbles. So I kept looking for better grain and finally discovered a knowledgeable lady that sold flour mills and who also was a serious baker herself. She had located a source of quality wheat with an assayed protein content and sold it by the 50 pound sack. When I asked her if her wheat was Organic she said it was either sixteen or seventeen percent protein depending on whether you wanted hard red spring wheat or hard white spring wheat. Organic or conventional? I persisted. No, she said. High protein!

So, I said to myself, since protein content is a function of soil fertility and since my body needs protein, I figured I am better off eating the best quality wheat, pesticide/herbicide residues (if there are any) be damned. Think about it! The difference between seventeen percent and fourteen percent protein is about 25 percent. That percentage difference is the key threshold of nutritional deficiency that makes teeth fall out. We can't afford to accept 25% degradations in our nutritional quality in something that we eat every day and that forms the very basis of our dietary.

Please understand here that I am not saying that high protein wheats can't be grown organically. They certainly can. The founder of Great Harvest Bakery performs a valuable service locating and securing high-protein lots of organically grown wheats for his outlets. But often as not Organic products are no more nourishing than those grown with chemicals. Until the buyers at Organic whole food wholesalers get better educated about grain, obtaining one's personal milling stock from them will be a dicey proposition.

Sometimes Organic cereal can be far worse than conventional. To make a cereal Organic is a negative definition; if it hasn't had chemicals, then its Organic. Grain is one of the few foods that will still produce economic yields of low quality seed on extremely infertile soil or when half-smothered in weeds because herbicides weren't used for reasons of ideological purity. Vegetables will hardly produce anything under those conditions; carelessly grown fruits and vegetables are inevitably small, misshapen, unmarketable. But seed cleaning equipment can remove the contamination of weed seeds in cereal grains (at a cost.)

The price the farmer receives for Organic cereal grain is much higher, so it is possible to accept rather low yields or expend more money for cleaning out high levels of weed seeds from the field-run harvest, and still make a good profit. A lousy Organic cereal crop like this might even make a higher profit because the farmer has been spared the expense of fertilization, of rotation, of weed control. I remember once I bought a sack of Organic whole oats that were the smallest, most shriveled, bitterest oats I've ever tried to eat. We ended up throwing out that tiny, light (lacking density) seed in favor of using the "conventional" whole oats that were plump, heavy and sweet.

Wheat is not the only cereal that is damaged by industrial milling. So are oats. Most consumers have never seen whole oats; they look very much like wheat berries. But rolled oats become rancid and stale on the shelf much like wheat flour on the shelf.

Another pitfall about using whole grains is that to be nutritious they must still be fresh enough to sprout vigorously. A seed is a package of food surrounding an embryo. The living embryo is waiting for the right conditions (temperature and moisture) to begin sprouting. Sprouting means the embryo begins eating up stored food and making a plant out of it. All foods are damaged by exposure to oxygen, so to protect the embryo's food supply, the seed is surrounded by a virtually airtight seed coat that permits only enough oxygen to enter for the embryo's respiration (yes, seed breaths slowly). Often the embryo is located at the edge of the seed and has its own air intake port. When the seed coat is removed or damaged, the innards are exposed to air and begin deteriorating rapidly. In the case of oats, especially rapidly, because oats are the only grass-based cereal that contains large quantities of oil–five percent oil, more or less. That's why oats "stick to your ribs." Rolled oats become stale and lose their flavor (and nutritional content) and perhaps become rancid very rapidly. So we make porridge from whole oat groats that we coarsely grind to grits (steel-cut oats) in an electric seed/spice mill just before cooking.

It is not easy to cook oat grits. They take a lot longer than rolled oats and if not done exactly to the recipe I'm about to give you, will almost inevitably stick to the pot badly and may also froth over and mess the stove. Here's how to cook them. Coarsely grind (like corn meal) your whole oats until you have one cup of oat grits. Bring exactly four cups of water (no salt) to a very hard boil at your highest heat. You may add a handful of raisins. Light or turn on a second, small-sized burner on the stove and set it as low as possible. Into the fast boiling water, slowly pour the ground oats, stirring continuously. Take about 30 seconds to pour it all or you'll make clumps. Keep on the high heat until the water again boils vigorously. Suddenly, the mixture will begin rising in the pot and will try to pour all over the stove. This means it is all at boiling temperature again. Quickly move the pot to the low burner; that instantly stops the frothing. Then cover. Let the porridge cook for 30 minutes, stirring once or twice to prevent sticking. Then, keeping it covered, turn off the heat. They can be eaten at this point but I think it is better to let the oats finish soaking on the stove for at least two to four hours. Then reheat in a double boiler, or warm in a microwave.

We usually start a pot of oats at bedtime for the next morning. See why people prefer the convenience of using rolled oats? But once you've eaten oats made right, you'll never prefer the flavor of rolled oats again. And if the human body has any natural method of assaying nutritional content, it is flavor.

Nutritionally, millet is almost the same story as oats. Millet seed is protected by a very hard hull. Cooking unhulled millet is almost impossible. After hours of boiling the small round seeds will still be hard and the hulls remain entirely indigestible. Worse, the half-round hulls (they split eventually) stick in your teeth. But prehulled millet, sitting in the sack for weeks and months, loses a lot of nutrition and tastes very second-rate compared to freshly-hulled millet. It is possible to buy unhulled millet, usually by special order from the health food distributor—if you'll take a whole sack. Millet can be hulled at home in small batches. Here's how we figured out how to do it. There probably are better ways.

Using a cheap steel-burr flour mill, set the burrs just far enough apart that the seed is ground to grits, but not flour. This pops the hulls loose. An old mill with worn-out burrs works great for this job. Then you have to get some hand seed cleaning screens just large enough to pass the grits but not pass the hulls (most of them). Window screen or other hardware cloths won't work. Seed cleaning screens come in increments of 1/128 inch; we use a 6/64" round screen. Other batches of millet might work better with a screen one step larger or smaller. It will take you a little ingenuity to find hand-held screens. They're used by seed companies and farmers to clean small batches of seed for inspection and are usually about one square foot in size with a quality wooden frame. Larger frames made of the same screening material are used in big seed cleaning machines. (The hulls could also be winnowed out by repeatedly pouring the grit/hulls mixture back and forth between two buckets in a gentle breeze.)

After you've screened out most of the hulls, the rest will rinse out, floating off as you wash the grain prior to cooking. We never hull more than enough millet for two or three meals and keep the uncooked (unwashed) millet in the freezer in an airtight jar. It is interesting how people will accept poor nutrition and its consequent sickness as the price of convenience.

If you eat much buckwheat you should also figure out how to hull (sometimes called groating) it yourself. Someone should write a thorough book on the home milling of cereals. And perhaps sell the equipment by mail. Probably would be a good little homestead business.

Something else you need to keep in mind about seed. Even though the embryo's food supply is protected by the seed coat, it still slowly deteriorates, steadily oxidizing and losing nutritional value. Eventually old seed looses the ability to sprout. The decline in germination ability matches a decline in nutritional quality. Any seed you are going to use for eating should possess the ability to sprout, strongly and rapidly. (After you've comparatively sprouted a few grain samples, you'll know what I mean by this.) Fortunately, cereal grains usually sprout well for quite a few years after harvest if they have been stored cool and dry. Eating dead or near-dead seeds will help move you closer to the same condition yourself.

Finally, one more warning about buying store bread. Salt-free bread tastes "funny" to most people. It bakes fine, salt is not necessary to the leavening process, but no bakery could stay in business without salting their bread. The standard level of salt is two percent by weight. That is quite a lot! Two percent equals one teaspoonful per pound. I'll have more to say about the evils of salt later on.

I imagine some of my readers are feeling a little overwhelmed by all these warnings and "bewares ofs," and intricacies. They are used to taking no responsibility for securing their own food supply quality and have come to expect the "system" to protect them. I believe it is not because of lack of government intervention, but because of government intervention itself, our food system is very perverse. Until our mass consciousness changes, if you wish to make yourself and your family truly healthy, you are going to have to take charge and become quite a discriminating shopper. Unconscious consumers are on a rapid road to the total unconsciousness of death.

And again, let me remind you here that this one small book cannot contain everything you should know. The bibliography at the end of should become your guide to earning your post-graduate education in nutritional health.

Freshness *of* Fruits *&* Vegetables

Most people do not realize the crucial importance of freshness when it comes to produce. In the same way that seeds gradually die, fruits and vegetables go through a similar process as their nutritional content gradually oxidizes or is broken down by the vegetables own enzymes, but vegetables lose nutrition hundreds of times more rapidly than cereals. Produce was recently part of a living plant. It was connected to the vascular system of a plant and with few exceptions, is not intended by nature to remain intact after being cut. A lettuce or a zucchini was entirely alive at the moment of harvest, but from that point, its cells begin to die. Even if it is not yet attacked by bacteria, molds and fungi, its own internal enzymes have begun breaking down its own substances.

Vegetables, especially leafy vegetables, are far more critical in this respect than most ripe fruits. All, however, deteriorate much like radioactive material; they have a sort of half-life. The mineral content is stable, but in respect to the vitamins and enzymes and other complex organic components, each time period or "half life" results in the loss of half the nutrition. Suppose a lettuce has a half life of 48 hours, two days after harvest only 50 percent of the original nutrition remains. After two more days, half the remaining half is gone and only 25 percent is left. After two more days half of that 25 percent is lost. Thus six days after harvest and a lettuce contains only about 12 percent of its original nutrition. A two day half-life is only hypothetical. Those types of produce I classify as very perishable probably do have a half-life of from 36 to 48 hours. Moderately perishable produce has a half life of about 72 hours; durable types of produce have half lives of 96 hours or longer.

Vegetable Storage Potential		
Very Perishable	**Moderately Perishable**	**Durable**
lettuce	zucchini	apple
spinach	eggplant	squash
Chinese cabbage	sweet peppers	oranges
kale	broccoli	cabbage
endive	cauliflower	carrot
peaches	apricots	lemons
parsley		beets

The half life of produce can be lengthened by lowering its temperature. For that reason, sophisticated produce growers usually use hydrocooling. This process dumps a just-cut vegetable into icy water within minutes of being harvested, lowering core temperature to a few degrees above freezing almost immediately. When cut vegetables are crated up at field temperatures, and stacks of those crates are put in a cooler, it can take the inside of the stack 24 hours, or longer, to become chilled. Home gardeners should also practice hydrocooling. Fill your sink with cold water and wash/soak your harvest until it is thoroughly chilled before draining and refrigerating it. Or, harvest your garden early in the morning when temperatures are lowest.

Still, when you buy produce in the store it may have been sitting at room temperature for hours or possibly days.

The bottom line here: fresh is equally as important as unsprayed or organically grown!

The Real Truth *about* Salt *&* Sugar

First, let me remind certain food religionists: salt is salt is salt is salt and sugar is sugar is sugar. There are no good forms of salt and no good forms of sugar. Salt from a mine and salt from the sea both have the same harmful effect; white sugar, natural brown sugar, honey, molasses, corn syrup, maple syrup, whatever sweet have you. All are sugars and all have the similar harmful effects. I know of no harmless salt substitute that really tastes salty. Nutrisweet is basically harmless to most people and can be used as a very satisfactory replacement for sugars. A few people are unable to tolerate nutrisweet, causing the anti-chemicalists to circulate much anti-nutrisweet propaganda, but you should carefully consider this thought before dismissing nutrisweet–there is almost no food substance that some people are not allergic to or unable to digest. The fact that nutrisweet is made in a chemical vat and the fact that some cannot handle nutrisweet does not make it "of the devil."

And it's not all black and white with the other items either. Sea salt does have certain redeeming qualities not found in mined salt and under certain very special conditions, eating small quantities of salt may be acceptable. Similarly, some forms of sugar are not quite as harmful as other forms, though all are harmful.

The primary health problem caused by table salt is not that it contributes to high blood pressure in people with poor kidneys, though it does that. It is not that eating salt ruins the kidneys; salt probably does not do that. The real problem with salt is that sodium chloride is an adrenal stimulant, triggering the release of adrenal hormones, especially natural steroids that resist inflammation. When these hormones are at high levels in the blood, the person often feels very good, has a sense of well-being. Thus salt is a drug! And like many drugs of its type, salt is a habituating drug. However, we are so used to whipping our adrenals with salt that we don't notice it. What we do notice is that we think we like the taste of salted food and consider that food tastes flat without it. But take away a person's salt shaker and they become very uncomfortable. That's because the addict isn't getting their regular dose.

What's wrong with repetitive adrenal whipping is that adrenal fortitude is variable; many people's adrenals eventually fail to respond to the prod of salt and the body begins to suffer from a lack of adrenal hormones. Often those inheriting weak adrenals manifest semi-failure in childhood. The consequence is that ordinary, irritating substances begin causing severe irritation. The person becomes allergic to pollen, dust, foods, animal danders, etc. We see asthma, hay fever, sinusitis, etc. Though one can then discover specific allergens and try to remove them from the environment or diet, often this case can be solved far more easily by complete withdrawal from all salt. This rests the adrenals and they may recover their full function; almost certainly their function will improve. The asthma, allergies and etc., gradually vanish.

Most of us don't need to eat salt as a nutrient. There's enough sodium in one dill pickle to run a human body for a year. There's enough natural sodium in many types of vegetables to supply normal needs without using table salt. Perhaps athletes or other hard working people in the tropics eating deficient food grown on leached-out depleted soils, people that sweat buckets day after day may need a little extra sodium. Perhaps. Not having practiced in the humid tropics myself, I have no definitive answer about this.

Unfortunately, the average American is entirely addicted to salt and thinks food tastes lousy without it. To please the average consumer, almost all prepared foods contain far too much salt for someone suffering from exhausted adrenals. Interestingly, Canadians do not like their foods nearly as salty as Americans, and prepared foods like soups and the like in cans and packages that look just like the ones in American supermarkets (though with French on the back panel) have to be reformulated for our northern neighbors. I've observed that Canadians are generally healthier than Americans in many respects.

We would all be far better off consuming no salt at all. Those with allergies or asthma should completely eliminate it for a month or two and discover if that simple step doesn't pretty much cure them. The trouble is that bakery bread is routinely two percent salt by weight. Cheese is equally salted or even more so. Canned and frozen prepared food products are all heavily salted. Restaurant meals are always highly salted in the kitchen. If you want to avoid salt you almost have to prepare everything yourself, bake your own bread, abstain from cheese (though there are unsalted cheeses but even I don't like the flavor of these), and abstain from restaurants. My family has managed to eliminate all salt from our own kitchen except for that in cheese, and we eat cheese rather moderately.

Sugar is a high-caloric non-food with enormous liabilities. First, from the viewpoint of the universal formula for health, no form of non-artificial sweetener carries enough nutrients with it to justify the number of calories it contains, not even malt extract. White refined sugar contains absolutely no nutrients at all; the "good" or "natural" sweets also carry so little nutrition as to be next to useless. Sweets are so far over on the bad end of the Health = Nutrition / Calories scale that for this reason alone they should be avoided.

However, healthy people can usually afford a small amount of sin; why not make it sweets? In small quantity, sugars are probably the easiest indiscretion to digest and the least damaging to the organ systems. Although, speaking of sin, as Edgar Guest, the peoples' poet, once so wisely quipped, (and my husband agrees) "Candy is dandy, but liquor is quicker." Sugar is a powerful drug! People who abuse sweets set up a cycle of addiction that can be very hard to break. It starts when the body tries to regulate blood sugar. Kicked up to high levels by eating sugar, the pancreas releases insulin. But that is not the end of the chain reaction. Insulin regulates blood sugar levels but also raises brain levels of an amino acid called tryptophan. Tryptophan is the raw material the brain uses to manufacture a neurotransmitter called serotonin. And serotonin plays a huge role in regulating mood. Higher brain levels of serotonin create a feeling of well-being. Eating sugar gives a person a chemical jolt of happiness. Heavy hits of high-glycemic index starch foods are also rapidly converted to sugar. So don't give your kids sweets! Or huge servings of starch to mellow them out. It is wise not to start out life a happiness addict with a severe weight problem.

Now that the chemistry of sugar addiction is understood, there currently is a movement afoot to cast the obese as helpless victims of serotonin imbalances and to "treat" them with the same kinds of serotonin-increasing happy drugs (like Prozac) that are becoming so popular with the psychiatric set. This promises to be a multiple billion dollar business that will capture all the money currently flowing into other dieting systems and bring it right back to the AMA/drug company/FDA nexus. The pitch is that when serotonin levels are upped, the desire to eat drops and so is weight. This approach is popular with the obese because it requires no personal responsibility other than taking a pill that really does make them feel happy. However, the same benefit can be had by strict adherence to a low-fat, low-carbohydrate diet. Eventually, the brain chemistry rebalances itself and serotonin levels stabilize.

Glycemic Index
(compared to glucose, which is 100)

Grains		Fruits		Vegetables	
all bran	51	apples	39	baked beans	40
brown rice	66	bananas	62	beets	64
buckwheat	54	cherries	23	black-eyed peas	33
cornflakes	80	grapefruit	26	carrots	92
oatmeal	49	grapes	45	chic peas	36
shred. wheat	67	orange juice	46	parsnips	97
muesli	66	peach	29	potato chips	51
white rice	72	orange	40	baked potato	98
white spaghetti	50	pear	34	sweet potato	48
whole wheat spaghetti	42	plum	25	yams	51
sweet corn	59	raisins	64	peas	51
Nuts		**Baked Goods**		**Sugars**	
peanuts	13	pastry	59	fructose	20
		sponge cake	46	glucose	100
Meats		white bread	69	honey	87
sausage	28	w/w bread	72	maltose	110
fish sticks	38	whole rye bread	42	sucrose	59
Dairy Products					
yogurt	36	whole milk	34	skim milk	32

Remember, the pancreas has another major service to perform for the body: secreting digestive enzymes to aid in the digestion of proteins. When the diet contains either too much protein or too much sugar and/or high-glycemic index starch foods, the overworked pancreas begins to be less and less efficient at maintaining both of these functions.

Sometimes a stressed-out pancreas gets overactive and does too good a job lowering the blood sugar, producing hypoglycemia. Hypoglycemia is generally accompanied by unpleasant symptoms such as fatigue, dizziness, blurred vision, irritability, confusion, headache, etc. This condition is typically alleviated by yet another hit of sugar which builds an addiction not only to sugar, but to food in general. If the hypoglycemic then keeps on eating sugar to relieve the symptoms of sugar ingestion, eventually the pancreas becomes exhausted, producing an insulin deficiency, called diabetes. Medical doctors treat diabetes with insulin supplements either oral or intramuscular plus a careful diet with very low and measured amounts of sugar and starch for the remainder of the persons inevitably shortened and far less pleasant life. However, sometimes diabetes can be controlled with diet alone, though medical doctors have not had nearly as much success with this approach as talented naturopaths. Sometimes, long fasting can regenerate a pancreas. It is far better to avoid creating this disease!

The dietary management of hypoglycemia requires that not only refined but also unrefined sugars and starches with a high glycemic index be removed from the diet. (The glycemic index measures the ease with which the starch is converted into glucose in the body, and estimates the amount of insulin needed to balance it out.) This means no sugar, no honey, no white flour, no whole grains sweetened with honey, no sweet fruits such as watermelons, bananas, raisins, dates or figs. Potatoes are too readily converted into sugar. Jerusalem artichokes are a good substitute.

People with hypoglycemia can often control their symptoms with frequent small meals containing vegetable protein every two hours. When a non-sweet fruit is eaten such as an apple, it should be eaten with some almonds or other nut or seed that slows the absorption of fruit sugar. Hypoglycemics can improve their condition with vitamins and food supplements. See the next chapter.

Allergies to foods and environmental irritants are frequently triggered by low blood sugar. Mental conditions are also triggered by low blood sugar levels, frequently contributing to or causing a cycle of acting out behavior accompanied by destruction of property and interpersonal violence, as well as psychosis and bouts of depression. It is not possible to easily deal with the resulting behavior problems unless the hypoglycemia is controlled. Unfortunately most institutions such as mental hospitals and jails serve large amounts of sugar and starch and usually caffeinated beverages, with a high availability of soda pop, candy, and cigarettes at concessions. If the diet were drastically improved, the drugs given to control behavior in mental hospitals would be much more effective at a lower dose, or unnecessary.

The insulin-cycle overworked pancreas may eventually not be able to secrete enough enzymes to allow for the efficient digestion of foods high in protein. As stated earlier, poor protein digestion leads to a highly toxic condition from putrefied protein in the intestines. This condition is alleviated by eliminating animal proteins from the diet and taking digestive aids such as pancreatin pills with meals to assist in the digestion of vegetable proteins.

Food Combining & "Healthfood Junkfood"

This brings us to a topic I call healthfood junkfood. Many people improve their diet, eliminating meat and chemicalized food in favor of whole grains and organically grown foods, but they then proceed to make these otherwise good foods into virtual junkfood by preparing them incorrectly. In my travels, I've noticed this same thing happens everywhere on Earth. What should be health-producing dietaries are ruined by frying, salting and sugaring.

Healthfood junkfoods include organically grown potato chips deep fried in cold pressed organic unsaturated canola oil (made rancid by frying) sprinkled with natural sea salt; organically grown oat and nut granola roasted with cold-pressed unsaturated oil (made rancid by roasting) hideously sweetened with honey; carrot cake made with rancid whole wheat flour, cold pressed unsaturated oil (made rancid by baking), honey, and cream cheese (salted); whole wheat cookies (stale, rancid flour) sweetened with honey, made with vegetable oil baked at high heat (rancid); whole wheat pizza vegetarian style with lots of soy cheese; whole wheat pizza vegan style with lots of real raw milk cheese; organically grown corn chips deep fried in cold pressed vegetable oil with or without natural sea salt, yogurts made from powdered milk without an active culture of beneficial bacteria and covered with highly sugared fruits, etc. These foods may well represent an improvement over the average American diet, but they still are not healthy foods, and should never be used in a diet for a sick person. Nor are they worthy of a person attempting to maximize health.

The problem with healthfood junkfoods is not their major ingredients, but how they were combined and processed and adulterated. Remember, fats, animal or vegetable, subjected to high heat become indigestible and toxic and make anything they're cooked with indigestible; salt is a toxic drug; cheese, hard enough to digest as it is, when raised to high temperatures as it is when making pizza, becomes virtually indigestible and cheese inevitably contains a lot of butterfat which, though saturated animal fat, when raised to high temperatures, still becomes slightly rancid. And all these foods represent indigestible combinations.

My clients almost never believe me when I first explain the idea of food combining. They think if it goes in one end, comes out the other, and they don't feel any unpleasant symptoms in between, then it was digested. But bad food combinations have a cumulative degenerative effect over a long period of time. When the symptoms arrive the victim never associates the food combination with the symptom because it seems to them that they've always been eating the food.

Mainstream nutritionists have brainwashed the public into thinking that we should have a representative serving from each of the "four basic food groups" at each and every meal, plus a beverage and a desert. Or, as my husband Steve is fond of quipping, a "balanced meal" has four colors on every plate: something red, something green, something white and something yellow. But the balanced meal is a gastronomic catastrophe that can only be processed by the very young with high digestive vitality, the exceptionally vital of any age, people with cast iron stomachs which usually refers to their good heredity, and those who are very physically active.

Few seem to realize that each type of food requires specific and different digestive enzymes in the mouth, stomach, and intestine. Carbohydrates, fats, proteins—each requires differing acid or alkaline environments in order to be digested. Proteins require an acid environment. Starch digestion requires an alkaline environment. When foods in complex combinations are presented to the stomach all together, like a meal with meat, potatoes, gravy, vegetables, bread, butter, a glass of milk, plus a starchy sweet desert, followed by coffee or tea, the stomach, pancreas, liver and small intestine are overwhelmed, resulting in the fermentation of the sugars and starches, and the putrefaction of the proteins, and poor digestion of the whole. It is little wonder that most people feel so tired after a large meal and need several cups of strong coffee to be able to even get up from the table. They have just presented their digestive tract with an immensely difficult and for some an impossible task.

For the most efficient digestion, the body should be presented with one simple food at a time, the one bowl concept, easily achieved by adherence to the old saying, "one food at a meal is the ideal." An example of this approach would be eating fruits for breakfast, a plain cereal grain for lunch, and vegetables for supper. If you can't eat quite that simply, then proper food combining rules should be followed to minimize digestive difficulty, maximize the adsorption of nutrients from your food, and reduce or eliminate the formation of toxemia, and of course foul gas.

In general, fruit should be eaten alone unless you happen to be hypoglycemic or diabetic in which case fruit should be eaten with small quantities of a vegetable protein such as nuts, or yogurt and/or cheese if able to digest dairy. Starches should be eaten with vegetables, which means that a well combined meal would include a grain such as rice, millet, buckwheat, amaranth, quinoa, corn, wheat, rye, oats, spelt, potatoes, or starchy winter squash combined with raw or cooked vegetables. Protein foods such as meat, eggs, beans, lentils, tofu, split peas, should be combined with vegetables, raw or cooked. But protein should never be combined with starches. The most popular North

American snacks and meals always have a starch/protein combination, for example: meat and potatoes, hamburger in a bun, hot dog with bun, burrito with meat or cheese, meat sandwiches, etc. It is little wonder that intestinal gas is accepted as normal, and that over time these hard to digest combinations eventually cause health problems that demand attention.

Another sure fire way to ruin any food, including the very best available is to eat in the presence of negative emotions generated by yourself or others. Negative emotions include fear, anger, frustration, envy, resentment, etc. The digestive tract is immediately responsive to stress and or negative thoughts. It becomes paralyzed in negative emotional states; any foods eaten are poorly digested, causing toxemia.

It is natural for a person who has lost a loved one or suffered a great loss of any kind to lose their appetite for a period of time. This reaction is pro-survival, because while grieving, the body is gripped by powerful negative emotions. There are people who, under stress or when experiencing a loss, eat ravenously in an attempt to comfort themselves. If this goes on for long the person can expect to create a serious illness of some kind.

Individual sensitivity to this type of overeating is dependent upon genetics and personality and who is generating the negative emotions. Self generated negative emotions are very difficult to avoid. If you are unable to change your own emotional tone or that of others around you, then it is important to eat very lightly, eat only easily digested foods such as raw fruits and vegetables, raw juices, steamed vegetables, and small servings of whole grains, nuts and seeds.

Diets *to* Heal *the* Critically Ill

A critically ill person is someone who could expire at any moment; therapeutic interventions are racing against death. Can the body repair itself enough before some essential function ceases altogether? If there already exists too much damage to vital organs the person will die. If there remains sufficient organ function to support life, enough vital force to power those functions, and a will to live, the body may heal itself if helped by the correct therapeutic approach. But the therapy does not do the healing; the body does that by itself–if it can. This reality is also true of allopathic medicine.

I believe fasting is the therapy that almost invariably gives a critically ill person their very best chance of recovery. If a patient dies while fasting they almost certainly would have died anyway, and if death comes while fasting, it will be more comfortable, with less pain, and with more mental clarity.

Critically ill people may have, among other things, any of the following diagnoses: advanced cancer, advanced aids, heart failure, very high blood pressure, kidney failure, advanced liver disease, advanced emphysema, pneumonia or other catastrophic infections, especially those that seem unresponsive to antibiotics, strokes, emboli, sclerotic vessels as found in arteriosclerosis, severe nerve degeneration interfering with nerve transmission to vital organs.

Treating the critically ill does not have to be an all or nothing, ideological choice between holistic medicine and AMA style medicine. It is important for the critically ill and their families to know that if they use standard medical treatment such as drugs or surgery, these measures can and should be combined with natural healing methods. It is always desirable to quit all addicting substances, start a whole foods diet, (as light as possible), and add meganutrition (supplements) to the medical doctor's treatments. Few medical doctors are so arrogantly partisan as to assert that natural measures will do any harm as long as the MD is still allowed to prescribe as they please.

Holistic support will not only lessen the side effects of the medical treatments but will speed up healing and often reduce the required dose of prescribed drugs. I have had several clients with cancer who chose to have surgery, radiation and chemotherapy, but stayed on a raw food diet and took high doses of supplements throughout the treatment. These people amazed the attending physician by feeling good with little if any fatigue, no hair loss, or flu symptoms. The same can be true of other conditions.

Food In The Order Of Digestive Difficulty

Individual digestive weaknesses and allergies are not taken into account in this list.

Hard To Digest: Meat, fish, chicken, eggs (if cooked), all legumes including soy products, peanuts and peanut butter, beans, split peas, lentils, chick peas, dairy products such as cheese, milk, butter milk, nuts and seeds and their butters.

Intermediate: all grains—quinoa, amaranth, millet, spelt, rye, wheat, oats, barley.

Fairly Easy: Brussels sprouts, green beans, green peas, broccoli, cauliflower, raw cultured milk products, asparagus, cabbage, sprouts especially bean sprouts, kale, other leafy greens.

Very Easy: fruits, vegetable juices, fruit juices, broth (clear).

No Effort: herb tea, water.

Ethyl always comes to my mind when I think of how much healing power can still be left in a dying body. She (accompanied by her husband for support) came to Great Oaks School with terminal cancer, heart failure, advanced diabetes, extreme weakness, and complete inability to digest. Any food ingested just came back up immediately. Ethyl had large tumors taking over the breast, sticking out from her skull, and protruding from her body in general. The largest was the one in the left breast which was the size of a big man's fist.

She did have one crucial thing going for her, Ethyl was a feisty Irish red head who still had a will to live, and a reason to do so. She and her husband, who had just retired, had dreamed their whole life of touring the US and Canada in their own RV the minute he retired. The time had finally arrived but Ethyl was too ill to support her own weight (only 90 pounds) and to top it off was blind from diabetic retinopathy. The doctors had done everything they could to her, and now judged her too weak to withstand any more surgery (she had already had her right breast removed). Radiation or chemotherapy were also considered impossible due to heart failure. They sent Ethyl home to die, giving her a few days to a month at most.

Any sensible hygienist trying to stay out of jail would have refused to take on this type of case because it was a cancer case where death was likely. Treatment of this highly lucrative disease is considered the AMA's exclusive franchise, even when the medical doctors have given up after having done everything to a body the family can pay for or owe for. Whenever a person dies under the care of any person who is not a licensed M.D. there must be an autopsy and a criminal investigation in search of negligence. If the person dies under the care of an M.D. the sheriff's assumption is that the doctor most assuredly did everything he could and should have done and death was inevitable. By accepting Ethyl I had a reasonable likelihood of ending up in trouble; but being foolish, brave and (stupidly) feeling relatively immune to such consequences (I was under 40 at the time), it seemed important to try to help her. So, undaunted by the task, regardless of the outcome, I proceeded logically, one step at a time. Today, with more experience and a modest net worth I wouldn't want to have to defend in a lawsuit, and at age 55. possessing no spare five to ten years to give to the State to "pay" for my bravery, I would probably refuse such a case. Fortunately I have not been confronted with this problem lately.

Since Ethyl was unable to digest anything given by mouth, she was fed rectally with wheat grass juice implants three times a day. She was carried to the colonic table for a daily colonic. Wheat grass and clay poultices were applied to her tumors three times a day. She received an acupressure massage and reflexology treatments during the day, plus a lot of tender loving care. This program continued for a month during which the tumors were being reabsorbed by the body, including the large, extremely hard tumor sticking out the flesh of the right breast.

Ethyl complained of severe pain as the large tumor in her breast shrank. While it had been getting larger and pressing ever harder on all the nerves, she had little or no sensation, but as it shrank, the nerves were reactivated. Most people think that a growing tumor would cause more pain than a shrinking one. Often the opposite is true. Pain can be a good sign that the body is winning, an indicator to proceed.

By the second month, Ethyl, gradually gaining strength, was able to take wheat grass and carrot juice orally, and gradually eased into raw foods, mostly sprouts and leafy greens such as sunflower and buckwheat greens grown in trays. She started to walk with assistance up and down the halls, no longer experiencing the intense pain formerly caused by a failing heart, and most surprising of all, her eyesight returned, at first seeing only outlines, and then details.

The third month Ethyl enlarged her food intake to include raw foods as well as the carrot and wheat grass juice and sprouts, plus vitamin and mineral supplements to help support her immune system and the healing process. All the tumors had been reabsorbed by her body and were no longer visible, her heart was able to support normal activity such as walking, and non-strenuous household chores, and her diabetes had corrected itself to the point that she no longer required insulin and was able to control her blood sugar with diet.

Her husband was then instructed in her maintenance and they went home to continue the program. The last I heard from them they had made two lengthy trips around the US in their RV and were enjoying their retirement together after all.

My treatment worked because the most important factor in the healing of the critically ill person is not give them more nourishment than their body is able to process. The moment the digestive capacity of the sick person is exceeded, the condition will be exacerbated and in a critically illness, the person is likely to die. If the body still has sufficient organ integrity and vital force to heal itself, it will do so only if given the least possible nourishment that will support life–provided no essential organs are hopelessly damaged. If the liver and kidneys are functional, and the person has done some previous dietary improvement and/or cleansing, success is likely, especially if the person wants to live.

A person in critical condition does not have time to ease into fasting by first spending a month or two on a raw foods diet. This means that the person who is taking care of the critically ill person must be experienced enough to adjust the intensity of the body's healing efforts and accurately assess the ability of the person to process toxic waste products clamoring for removal so the ailing body is not drowned in it's own poisons. It is often necessary to use clear vegetable broth, vegetable and wheat grass juices, and fruits juices, or whole sprouts to slow down the cleansing gradient and sometimes, to resupply the tissue's exhausted nutritional reserves.

I wish all cases of critical illness had such a positive outcome as Ethyl's, but unfortunately they don't. I had Marge on the same program at the same time. She also had cancerous tumors all over her body and had similarly been sent home to die. In some ways Marge's body was a more likely candidate for survival than Ethyl's. Marge did not have heart failure or diabetes and was still able on arrival to at least take small amount of water orally and walk to the bathroom. Put on a similar program, her tumors also shrunk and were reabsorbed and she too went home.

But Marge did not really have a strong reason to live. Although her husband was by her side throughout the treatment program, Marge was deeply upset because she was estranged from one of her sons who she had not seen for over 10 years. When she went home from Great Oaks, the son finally consented to see his mother, went to the effort of trying to work things out with her, and finally confessed that under it all he still loved her.

At that point Marge died in peace. She had accomplished the last thing she wanted to take care of and her will to live did not extend beyond that point. Had she died several months earlier as predicted by the medical profession, Marge would have been unable to resolve this relationship. This was what Marge's life was pivoting on at the end. I was glad to assist her in doing what she needed to do. Her husband and other family members found it difficult to understand, and they were hurt that Marge did not wish to continue her life with them.

Diet *for the* Chronically Ill

The chronically ill person has a long-term degenerative condition that is not immediately life threatening. This condition usually causes more-or-less continuous symptoms that are painful, perhaps unsightly, and ultimately will be disabling or eventually capable of causing death. To qualify as "chronic" the symptoms must have been present a minimum of six months, with no relief in sight. People with these conditions have usually sought medical assistance, frequently have had surgery, and have taken and probably are taking numerous prescription drugs.

Some examples of chronic conditions are: arthritis, rheumatism, diabetes, early onset of cancer and aids, asthma, colitis, diverticulitis, irritable bowel syndrome, some mental disorders, arterial deposit diseases, most of the itises (inflammations).

Before fasting, the chronically ill often do have time to prepare the way with limited dietary reform, and frequently begin to feel relief quite quickly. Before actually fasting they should limit their diet to raw foods and eliminate all toxic foods like alcohol, coffee, tea, salt, sugar and recreational drugs for two months if they have been following a typical American diet.

If the chronically ill had been following a vegetarian diet, perhaps a diet including with eggs and dairy, if they had been using no addicting substances, then one month on raw foods is sufficient preparation for fasting. If the person had water or juice fasted for at least a week or two within the last two years, and followed a healthy diet since that time, one or two weeks on raw foods should be a sufficient runway.

During preparation for a fast, I never recommend that a chronically ill person quit taking prescription medicines because doing so can seriously disrupt their homeostasis. However, if their symptoms lessen or vanish during the pre-fasting clean up, the person might try tapering off medications.

The length and type of fast chosen to resolve a chronic illness depends largely on available time, finances, availability of support people, work responsibilities, and mental toughness. If you are one of those fortunate people 'rich' enough to give their health first priority, long water fasting is ideal. If on the other hand you can't afford to stop working, have no one to take care of you and assist with some household chores, and/or you are not mentally tough enough to deal with self-denial, compromise is necessary.

Ideally the chronically ill person would fast for an extended period under supervision until their symptoms were gone or greatly improved, with a fall-back plan to repeat the whole process again in three to six months if necessary. If you are not able to do that, the next best program is to fast for a short period, like one or two weeks, with a plan to repeat the process as often as possible until you are healed.

I have had clients with potentially life-threatening conditions such as obesity with incipient heart failure, or who came to me with cancer, that were unable to stop work for financial reasons, or who could not afford a residential fasting program, or who felt confident in their own ability to deal with detoxification in their own home. These people have fasted successfully at home, coming to see me once a week. Almost inevitably, successful at-home fasters had already done a lot of research on self healing, believed in it, and had the personal discipline to carry it out properly, including breaking the fast properly without overeating.

Foods To Heal Chronic Illness

Sprouts	Baby Greens	Salad	Juices	Fruit
alfalfa	sunflower	lettuce	beet	grapefruit
radish	buckwheat	celery	celery	lemon
bean	zucchini	zucchini	lime	lime
clover	kale	kale	orange	orange
fenugreek	endive	radish	parsley	apple
wheat		tomato	tomato	raspberries
cabbage		cabbage	cabbage	blueberries
		carrot	carrot	grapes
		spinach	apple	peaches
		parsley	grapefruit	apricots
		sweet pepper	lemon	strawberry

Fruits should be watery and lower in sugar. Some examples of poor fruit choices would be pineapple, ripe mango, bananas, dates, raisins, figs. Fruits should not be combined with vegetables.

Vegetables should not be starchy, packed-full of energy. Poor vegetable choices would be potato, parsnip, turnip, corn, sweet potato, yam, beet, winter squash. Sprouts and baby greens are vegetables and may be included in salads.

Juices should not be extremely sweet. Apple, orange, beet and carrot juice should be diluted with 50% water. Fruit juices should not be mixed with vegetable juices or with vegetables at the same meal.

Salads should include no fruit. Salad dressings should be lemon or lime juice, very small quantities of olive oil, and herbs. No salt, soy sauce nor black pepper. Cayenne can be okay for some.

I have also helped chronically ill people that were not mentally prepared to water fast, but were able to face the long-term self-control and deprivation of a raw food cleansing diet that included careful food combining. These people also regained their health, but it took them a year at minimum, and once well they had to remain on a diet tailor-made to their digestive capacity for the rest of their life, usually along with food supplements.

Jim was such a case. He was 55 years old, very obese, had dangerously high blood pressure poorly controlled with medication, and was going into congestive heart failure. He was on digitalis and several other heart medications plus diuretics, but in no way was his condition under control. He had severe edema in the feet and legs with pitting, and fluid retention in the abdominal region caused a huge paunch that was solid to the touch not soft and squishy like fatty tissue.

Jim had dreamed of having his own homestead with an Organic garden, now he had these things but was too sick to enjoy them or work in his garden without severe heart pain and shortness of breath. Jim had retired early in order to enjoy many years without the stresses of work, and he was alarmed to realize that he was unlikely to survive a year.

The day Jim came to see me the first time I would have classified his condition as critically ill because his life was in immediate danger; but he responded so quickly to his detox program that he was very soon out of danger and would be more accurately described as a chronically ill person. Jim was not prepared to water fast. He was attached to having his food and he was aware that at his extreme weight he was going to have stay on a dietary program for a long, long time. He also wanted to choose a gradient that he could manage by himself at home with little assistance from his wife. He had been on a typical American diet with meat, coffee, etc., so that in spite of his dangerous condition it did not seem wise to me to add the heavy eliminatory burden of a water fast to a body that was already overwhelmed with fluids and waste products.

Jim immediately went on a raw food cleansing diet, with no concentrated foods like nuts, seeds, or avocados, and with one day each week fasting on vegetable juice and broth. He did enemas daily even though it wasn't his favorite thing. In one month he had lost 30 pounds, his eyes had started to sparkle, and his complexion was rosy. The swelling had disappeared from his feet and legs, and he had to buy new pants.

Starting the second month he gradually withdrew from prescription medications. From the beginning I had put Jim on a program of nutritional supplements including protomorphogens (see chapter on vitamins and food supplements) to help the body repair it's heart and the kidneys. In only four months he had returned his body to glowing health, and looked great for his age, though he was still overweight. At the end of one year he had returned to a normal weight for his height, and only cheated on the diet a couple of times when attending a social event, and then it was only a baked potato with no dressing.

He was probably going to have many qualitative years working his garden and living out his dreams. The local intensive care ward lost a lot of money when they failed to get Jim.

Diet *for the* Acutely Ill

The acutely ill person experiences occasional attacks of distressing symptoms, usually after indiscretions in living or emotional upsets. They have a cold, or a flu, or sinusitis, or a first bout of pneumonia, or a spring allergy attack. The intense symptoms knock them flat and force them to bed for a few days or a week. If they are sick more often than that, they are moving toward the chronically ill category.

People who are acutely ill should stop eating to whatever extent that they are able until the symptoms are gone. During an acute illness, the appetites is probably pretty dull anyway, so why not give a brief fast on water or fruit juice a try.

Most acute conditions are short in duration, usually not lasting more than a week. Allergy attacks, some types of flu, and a first bout of pneumonia may well last for three weeks or a month. The general rule is to eat as little as possible until the symptoms have passed, self-administer colon cleansing, even if you have a horror of such things, and take vitamin supplements, including megadoses of Vitamin C, bioflavinoids, and zinc. (See the chapter on vitamins.) Those having a little experience with natural medicine make teas of echinacea, fenugreek seeds and red clover and quit eating. Eating as little as possible can mean only water and herb teas, only vegetable broth, only vegetable juice or non-sweet fruit juice, even only cleansing raw foods. If you eat more than this you have not relieved your system of enough digestive effort.

After your symptoms are gone it is very important to change your life-style and improve your diet so that you aren't so toxic and don't have to experience an acute illness several times a year when your body is forced to try an energetic detox.

Diet *for a* Healthy Person

I doubt that it is possible to be totally healthy in the twentieth century. Doctors Alsleben and Shute in their book How to Survive the New Health Catastrophes state that in-depth laboratory testing of the population at large demonstrated four universally present pathological conditions: heavy metal poisoning, arteriosclerosis, sub-clinical infections, and vitamin/mineral deficiencies. Those of us who consider ourselves healthy, including young people, are not really healthy, and at the very least would benefit from nutritional supplementation. In fact the odds against most people receiving adequate vitamin and mineral nutrition without supplements are very poor as demonstrated by the following chart.

Problem Nutrients in America	
Nutrient	**Percent Receiving Less than the RDA**
B-6	80%
Magnesium	75
Calcium	68
Iron	57
Vitamin A	50
B-1	45
C	41
B-2	36
B-12	36
B-3	33

A genuinely healthy person almost never becomes acutely ill, and does not have any disturbing or distracting symptoms; nothing interferes with or handicaps their daily life or work. A healthy person has good energy most of the time, a positive state of mind, restful sleep, good digestion and elimination.

Healthy people do not have to live simon-pure lives to remain that way. Healthy people can afford 10% dietary indiscretions by calorie count–eating or drinking those things that they know are not good for them but that are fun to eat or are "recreational foods or beverages." Such "sinning" could mean a restaurant bash twice a month, having a pizza, French bread, beer or wine in moderation, ice cream, cookies, cake, turkey for festive occasions, etc. The key concept of responsible sinning is keeping within that ten percent limit.

A diet for a healthy person that wants to remain healthy should not exceed the digestive capacity of the individual, either in terms of quantity or quality. All foods that can not be efficiently digested should be removed from the regular diet and relegated to the "sin" category, including those you are allergic to and those for which you have inadequate digestive enzymes. I have encountered very few people that can efficiently digest cooked meat, chicken, or fish, but some can, and some can with the assistance of digestive enzyme supplements. In order to digest meats, the stomach must be sufficiently acid, there must be enough pepsin, pancreatin, and bile, etc., and the meat should be eaten on the extremely rare side (not pork), in small quantities (not more than five or six ounces), and not combined with anything except nonstarchy vegetables. If you must include meat in your dietary, it should represent a very small percentage of your total caloric intake, be eaten infrequently, with the bulk of the calories coming from complex carbohydrates such grains, legumes and nuts, as well as large quantities of vegetables and fruits.

The healthy person that wants to stay that way for many, years is advised to fast one day a week, to give the organs of elimination a chance to catch up on their internal housecleaning. If water fasting seems impossible, try a day of juicing it; if that is too rigorous, try a day on raw foods. A similar technique, though less beneficial than even a one day each week on raw foods, is delaying breaking your overnight fast for as long as possible each day. Try giving up breakfast altogether or postponing breaking your overnight fast, because from the time you stop eating at the end of one day to the time you start eating the next is actually a brief, detoxifying fast.

Eggs, milk, cheese and yogurt can be assimilated by some healthy people with or without digestive aids. It is possible to take lactase to break down the milk sugars for example; sometimes aids such as hydrochloric acid, pepsin, and pancreatin help. If you can buy it or are willing to make it raw milk yogurt containing lactobacillus bulgaris or acidophilus may be digested more readily, especially if it prepared from healthy cows or goats fed on unsprayed food, and served very fresh. Eggs should come from chickens that run around outside, eating weeds, and scratching bugs. The yokes of those eggs will be intense orange, not yellow. Few people these days have ever eaten a real egg. Surprisingly, for those of you who fear cholesterol, the healthy way to eat eggs is use just the raw yolk from fertile eggs. It is enjoyed by many people in a smoothie–fresh fruit blended up with water or milk. Eggs contain lecithin, a nutrient that naturally prevents the body from forming harmful fatty deposits in the arteries.

Sea weeds are a wonderful source of minerals and should be eaten in soups and salads. Other invaluable fortifying foods are algae of all kinds (such as chlorella and spirulina), lecithin, brewers yeast, and fresh bakers yeast. Many people have had very unpleasant experiences trying to eat living bakers yeast and so use brewers yeast instead. But brewers yeast is cooked and the proteins it contains are not nearly as assimilable as those in raw yeast. Raw yeast is so powerful, it feels like pep pills!

It takes a special technique to eat raw yeast because in the stomach and intestines the yeast does the job it is supposed to do: convert sugars into alcohol and carbon dioxide gas. The entire digestive tract then bloats with gas and the person will feel very uncomfortable for some time. However, raw yeast is a marvelous source of B vitamins and proteins and can make someone feel very energetic–if they know how to use it. The secret is to eat live yeast very first thing in the morning on an empty stomach and then, not eat anything at all for about two hours, giving the stomach acids and enzymes time to kill the yeasts and digest them before adding sugars from another meal. Some like to eat yeast in fresh cake form, buying it from a bakery. Others prefer dry granular baker's yeast blended with water into a sort of "shake." This is not a bad place to put your raw egg yoke either. If you need it sweetened to drink it, use an artificial or herbal sweetener like nutrisweet or stevia. Live yeast cannot consume milk sugars very well. So if you can handle dairy, try one or two tablespoons of granulated live yeast, an egg yoke and a little raw milk or yogurt, well whizzed.

Wheat germ is also a great, rich food, but is usually rancid unless it is taken out of the refrigerated display; unless it is refrigerated, in a dated package and fresh, don't eat it. Herb teas and roasted grain beverages are healthy beverages, along with mineral and distilled water avoiding where possible chlorinated and fluoridated water.

Diet Is Not Enough

Those isolated, long-lived peoples discovered by Weston A. Price had to do hard physical labor to eat, had to walk briskly up and down steep terrain to get anywhere. But today, few North Americans output very much physical energy in process of daily life or work. Not only cars, but all of our modern conveniences make it possible to live without ever breaking into a sweat. We pay for this ease; it costs us a significant degree of health.

Exercise has many benefits when combined with excellent nutrition. It creates an overall feeling of well-being that can not be created by diet alone. Exercising temporarily makes the heart beat faster, increasing blood circulation throughout the body right out to the tips of your fingers and toes. This short-term elevated flow of blood flow brings increased supplies of oxygen and nutrients to all parts of the body,

147

facilitating healing and repair. Without revving up your engine every day many of the body's systems never get the sludge burned out of them and never perform optimally.

Exercise also changes the metabolic rate so your body burns more calories–not only while you are exercising, but also for a 24 hour period following exercise. This maintains a healthful body weight into old age, or helps to lose weight. Most people find that exercise in moderation does not increase appetite, so that it is possible to consistently burn more calories in a day, and gradually reduce weight if that is desirable. It is necessary to burn 3,500 calories to lose a pound of weight. Most forms of exercise allow you to burn 300 to 600 calories per hour at a moderate pace which would be achieved by doubling the resting pulse. Without even considering the weight-loss benefit of achieving a raised metabolism, an hour of daily exercise continued for a week or two dependent upon the type of exercise and pace should lead to one pound of weight loss if the caloric intake is held constant.

The flip side of having a higher metabolism is rarely appreciated but is extremely important. Recall the basic equation of health: Health = Nutrition / Calories. Exercise permits a person to eat somewhat more while not gaining weight. If the food is nutrient rich, the body has a chance to extract more vitamins, more minerals, more amino acids. The person who remains slender by rigidly reducing their food intake to near starvation levels may lack vital, health-building nutrition.

And only exercise moves lymphatic fluid. The blood is pumped through the body by the heart, but the lymphatic system, lacking a heart, requires muscular contractions to move from the extremities of the body to the central cavity. The lymphatic system picks up cellular waste products and conducts these toxins to disposal. Frequently, people with rheumatic aches and pains or other generalized muscular discomforts physicians like to give Latin diagnostic names to can give up taking pain pills if they will but begin exercising regularly. Only when they begin moving their lymph can they begin to detoxify properly.

There is another benefit from exercise which is not to be ignored, and that is that it gives the person a chemical sense of well being. It actually will help to emotionally boost up people who are chronically depressed and make them smile. After a good workout, especially one done outside, everything seems brighter, more positive; whatever was bothering you somehow just doesn't seem like that big of a deal now. I am not making pro-exercise propaganda. This is not a figment of the imagination. An exercising body really does make antidepressant neurochemicals called endorphins, but only after about 45 minutes to an hour of aerobic workout.

Endorphins are powerful, with painkilling and euphoric effects equal to or greater than heroin, but without any undesirable side effects. If chemists could learn to cheaply synthesize endorphins I'm sure that millions of people would want to become addicted to them. Because I make such a point of getting in my workout every day, my husband has accused me of being an endorphin junkie, and he is right! I admit it, I'm really hooked on the feeling of well being I consistently get from any sustained exercise. I defend my addiction staunchly because it is the healthiest addiction I know of.

I have also been accused of carrying exercise to extremes, and I admit to that also. For a few years I trained for Ironman triathlons. I now think doing ironman distances is immoderate and except for a few remarkable individuals with "iron" constitutions, training that hard can only lead to a form of exhaustion that is not health promoting. I have become much more sensible in my "old" age, and in recent years have limited my participation to the Olympic distance triathlons. I was on the Canadian team at the World Championship in 1992, and intend to do it again in 1995. I do not find the Olympic distance exhausting, in fact I think it is great fun and truly exhilarating. I get to see all these wonderful age group competitors from all over the world who look and feel fantastic. It does my soul good to see a group of people aging so gracefully, not buying into the popular notion that old age is inevitably disabling, depressing, and ugly. Sport brings a degree of balance to my life after spending so much time in the presence of the sick. I plan to maintain my athletic activities into old age, barring accident or other unforeseen obstacles to fitness.

To maintain basic fitness it does not matter so much what form of exercise is chosen, as long as it is not damaging to the skeletal system or connective tissues. Many people are unable to run due to foot, knee, hip, or back problems, but almost everyone can walk. Walking outside is better than inside on a treadmill, and walking hills is better than walking on flat ground. Exercise machines such as stationary bikes, cross country ski machines, and stair steppers work well for a lot of people who live in the city, especially in the winter, or for those who hate exercise. Whatever you choose to do, it is important to at least double the resting pulse for 30 minutes no less than four days a week. This is the absolute minimum required to maintain the health and function of the cardiovascular-pulmonary system. If your resting pulse is 70, you must walk, jog, ski, bike, swim or what have you, fast enough to keep the pulse at 140 beats per minute for at least 30 minutes.

I have a strong preference to exercising outside in isolated places where there is only me and the forest, or only me and the river. Running along logging roads in the hilly back country, or swimming in the green unpolluted water of a forest river is a spiritual experience for me. It is a time to meditate, to commune with nature, and to clear my mind and create new solutions. The repetitive action of running or walking or swimming, along with the regular deep breathing in clean air, with no distractions except what nature provides is truly health promoting. Sharing these activities with friends or family can also be great fun and some of the best in social interactions. It is one of my favorite ways of visiting with people. I don't expect other people to be as enthusiastic about exercise as I am, but I do hope that everyone will make an effort to be minimally fit as an ongoing part of their health program into old age.

Diet *for A* Long, Long Life

Some people not only want to be healthy, but they want to live in good health long past the normal life span projected by statistical tables for Homo Sapiens. Dr. Roy Walford, a well-respected medical research gerontologist who has been actively studying longevity for many years, is one of those. He has scientifically demonstrated with accepted studies that a qualitative life span up to at least 115 years of age is reasonably attainable by the average person if they start working on it no later than about 50 years of age, though earlier is much better.

Walford's principles of extending life are very simple. All you have to do is restrict your caloric intake to about 1,500 per day, and water fast two days a week. Or alternatively, reduce your caloric intake to 1,200 per day and fast only one day a week on water. And make sure that every single bit of food you do eat is packed with nutrition, every single calorie, without exception. You continue this program for the rest of your life along with moderate daily exercise and high but reasonable dosages of vitamins, minerals, and also take a few exotic food supplements. The supplement program is not particularly expensive nor extreme, Walford's supplement program is more moderate than the life extension program I recommend for all middle-aged and older people. The best foods for this type of program is a largely raw food diet (80%) with a predominance of sprouts and baby greens, some cooked vegetables, and raw nuts and seeds. And make sure you get 30 minutes of cardiovascular exercise every other day.

While Dr. Walford's focus is on caloric reduction while maintaining sufficient nutrition, most other life extensionists focus on increasing the nutrition side of the equation for health without bothering to reduce caloric intake. This approach is much easier because essentially, it involves gobbling nutritional supplements by the handfuls without requiring self-discipline, though it can get quite expensive. I'll have more to say about this approach in the next chapter, which is about vitamins.

In this book I can't explain all the aspects of prolongation of life through conscious life-style choice. Those who are interested are referred to the Bibliography.

Chapter Six

Vitamins & Other Food Supplements

From The Hygienic Dictionary

Vitamins. [1] The staple foods may not contain the same nutritive substances as in former times. . . . Chemical fertilizers, by increasing the abundance of the crops without replacing all the exhausted elements of the soil, may have indirectly contributed to change the nutritive value of cereal grains and of vegetables. . . . Hygienists have not paid sufficient attention to the genesis of diseases. Their studies of conditions of life and diet, and of their effects on the physiological and mental state of modern man are superficial, incomplete, and of too short duration. They have, thus, contributed to the weakening of our body and our soul. *Alexis Carrel, Man the Unknown.*

I have already explained the hygienist's view of why people get sick. The sequence of causation goes: enervation, toxemia, alternative elimination, disease. However, there is one more link in this chain, a precursor to enervation that, for good and understandable reasons, seemed unknown to the earlier hygienists. That precursor is long term sub-clinical malnutrition. Lack of nutrition effects virtually everybody today. Almost all of us are overfed but undernourished.

I have already explained that one particular head of broccoli does not necessarily equal another head of broccoli; the nutritional composition of apparently identical foods can be highly variable. Not only do different samples of the same type of food differ wildly in protein content, amino acid ratios and mineral content, their vitamin and vitamin-like substances also vary according to soil fertility and the variety grown.

These days, food crop varieties are bred for yield and other commercial considerations, such as shipability, storage life, and ease of processing. In pre-industrial times when each family propagated its own unique open-pollinated varieties, a natural selection process for healthy outcomes prevailed. If the family's particular, unique varieties carried genes for highly nutritious food, and if the family's land was fertile enough to allow those genes to manifest, and if the family kept up its land's fertility by wise management, their children tended to survive the gauntlet of childhood illness and lived to propagate the family's varieties and continue the family name. Thus, over time, human food cultivars were selected for their nutritional content.

But not any longer! These days, farming technology with its focus on bulk yield and profit, degrades the nutritional content of our entire food supply. Even commercial organically grown food is no better in this respect.

Sub-clinical, life-long, vitamin and mineral deficiencies contribute to the onset of disease; the malnourished body becomes increasingly enervated, beginning the process of disease. Vitamin supplements can increase the body's vital force, reversing to a degree the natural tendency towards degeneration. In fact, some medical gerontologists theorize that by using vitamins it might be possible to restore human life span to its genetically programmed 115 years without doing anything else about increasing nutrition from our degraded foods or paying much attention to dietary indiscretions. Knowing what I do about toxemia's effects I doubt vitamins can allow us to totally ignore what we eat, though supplements can certainly help.

More than degraded nutritional content of food prompts a thinking person to use food supplements. Our bodies and spirits are constantly assaulted and insulted by modern life in ways our genetics never intended us to deal with. Today the entire environment is mildly toxic. Air is polluted; water is polluted; our food supply contains traces of highly poisonous artificial molecules that our bodies have no natural ability to process and eliminate. Our cities and work places are full of loud, shocking noises that trigger frequent adrenaline rushes and other stress adaptations. Our work places are full of psychological stresses that humans never had to deal with before.

Historically, humans who were not enslaved have been in control of determining their own hour to hour, day to day activities, living on their own largely self-sufficient farms. The idea of working for another, at regular hours, without personal liberty, ignoring or suppressing one's own agenda and inclinations over an entire lifetime is quite new and not at all healthy. It takes continual subconscious applications of mental and psychic energies to protect ourselves against the stresses of modern life, energies that we don't know we're expending. This is also highly enervating. Thus to remain healthy we may need nutrition at levels far higher than might be possible through eating food; even ideal food might not contain enough vitamins to sustain us against the strains and stresses of this century.

And think about Dr. Pottenger's cats. Our bodies are at the poorer end of a century-long process of mass degeneration that started with white flour from the roller mill. Compared to my older clients I have noticed that my younger patients seem to possess less vital force on the average, show evidence of poorer skeletal development, have poorer teeth, less energy, have far more difficulty breeding and coping with their family life, and are far more likely to develop degenerative conditions early. Most of my younger patients had a poor start because they were raised on highly refined, devitalized, deficient foods, and grew up without much exercise. Their parents had somewhat better food. Some of their grandparents may have even grown up on raw milk and a vegetable garden, and actually had to walk, not owning cars when they were young. Their great grandparents had a high likelihood of enjoying decent nutrition and a healthful life-style.

Unfortunately, most of my patients like the idea of taking vitamins too much for their own good. The AMA medical model has conditioned people to swallow something for every little discomfort, and taking a pill is also by far the easiest thing to do because a pill requires no life-style changes, nor self-discipline, nor personal responsibility. But vitamins are much more frugal than drugs. Compared to prescriptions, even the most exotic life extension supplements are much less expensive. I am saddened when my clients tell me they can't afford supplements. When their MD prescribes a medicine that costs many times more they never have trouble finding the money.

I am also saddened that people are so willing to take supplements, because I can usually do a lot more to genuinely help their bodies heal with dietary modification and detoxification. Of all the tools at my disposal that help people heal, last in the race comes supplements.

One of the best aspects of using vitamins as though they were healing agents is that food supplements almost never have harmful side effects, even when they are taken in what might seem enormous overdoses. If someone with a health condition reads or hears about some vitamin being curative, goes out and buys some and takes it, they will at very least have followed the basic principle of good medicine: first of all do no harm. At worst, if the supplements did nothing for them at all, they are practicing the same kind of benevolent medicine that Dr. Jennings did almost two centuries ago. Not only that, but having done something to treat their symptoms, they have become patients facilitating their own patience, giving their body a chance to correct its problem. They well may get better, but not because of the action of the particular vitamin they took. Or, luckily, the vitamin or vitamins they take may have been just what was needed, raising their body's vital force and accelerating the body's ability to solve its problem.

One reason vitamin therapies frequently do not work as well as they might is that, having been intimidated by AMA propaganda that has created largely false fears in the public mind about harmful effects of vitamin overdoses, the person may not take enough of the right vitamin. The minimum daily requirements of vitamins and minerals as outlined in nutrition texts are only sufficient to prevent the most obvious forms of deficiency diseases. If a person takes supplements at or near the minimum daily requirement (the dose recommended by the FDA as being 'generally recognized as safe') they should not expect to see any therapeutic effect unless they have scurvy, beri beri, rickets, goiter, or pellagra.

In these days of vitamin-fortified bread and iodized salt, and even vitamin C fortified soft drinks, you almost never see the kind of life-threatening deficiency states people first learned to recognize, such as scurvy. Sailors on long sea voyages used to develop a debilitating form of vitamin C deficiency that could kill. Scurvy could be quickly cured by as little as one lime a day. For this reason the British Government legislated the carrying of limes on long voyages and today that is why British sailors are still called limeys. A lime has less than 30 milligrams of vitamin C. But to make a cold clear up faster with vitamin C a mere 30 mg does absolutely nothing! To begin to dent an infection with vitamin C takes 10,000 milligrams a day, and to make a life threatening infection like pneumonia go away faster might require 25,000 to 150,000 milligrams of vitamin C daily, administered intravenously. In terms of supplying that much C with limes, that's 300 to 750 of them daily—clearly impossible.

Similarly, pellagra can be cured with a few milligrams of vitamin B3, but schizophrenia can sometimes be cured with 3,000 milligrams, roughly a thousand times as much as the MDR.

There are many common diseases that the medical profession does not see as being caused by vitamin deficiencies. Senility and many mental disorders fall in this category. Many old people live on extremely deficient diets comprised largely of devitalized starches, sugars, and fats, partly because many do not have good enough teeth to chew vegetables and other high roughage foods, and they do not have the energy it takes to prepare more nourishing foods. Virtually all old people have deficiency diseases. As vital force inevitably declines with age, the quantity and quality of digestive enzymes decreases, then the ability to breakdown and extract soluble nutrients from food is diminished, frequently leading to serious deficiencies. These deficiencies are inevitably misdiagnosed as disease and as aging.

Suppose a body needs 30 milligrams a day of niacin to not develop pellagra, but to be fully healthy, needs 500 milligrams daily. If that body receives 50 milligrams per day from a vitamin pill, to the medical doctor it could not possibly be deficient in this vitamin. However, over time, the insidious sub-clinical deficiency may degrade some other system and produce a different disease, such as colitis. But the medical doctor sees no relationship. Let me give you an actual example. Medical researchers studying vitamin B5 or pantothenic acid noticed that it could, in what seemed to be megadoses (compared to the minimum daily requirement) largely reverse certain degenerative effects of aging. These researchers were measuring endurance in rats as it decreased through the aging process. How they made this measurement may appear to some readers to be heartless, but the best way to gauge the endurance of a rat is to toss it into a five gallon bucket of cold water and see how long it swims before it drowns. Under these conditions, the researcher can be absolutely confident that the rat does its very best to stay alive.

Young healthy rats can swim for 45 minutes in 50 degree Fahrenheit water before drowning. Old rats can only last about 15 minutes. And old rats swim differently, less efficiently, with their lower bodies more or less vertical, sort of dog paddling. But when old rats were fed pantothenic acid at a very high dose for a few weeks before the test, they swam 45 minutes too. And swam more efficiently, like the young rats did. More interestingly, their coats changed color (the gray went away) and improved in texture; they began to appear like young rats. And the rats on megadoses of B5 lived lot longer– 25 to 33 percent longer than rats not on large doses of B5. Does that mean "megadoses" of B5 have an unknown drug-like effect? Or does that mean the real nutritional requirement for B5 is a lot higher than most people think? I believe the second choice is correct. To give you an idea of how much B5 the old rats were given in human terms, the FDA says the minimum daily requirement for B5 is about 10 milligrams but if humans took as much B5 as the rats, they would take about 750 milligrams per day. Incidentally, I figure I am as worthy as any lab rat and take over 500 milligrams daily.

My point is that there is a big difference between preventing a gross vitamin deficiency disease, and using vitamins to create optimum functioning. Any sick person or anyone with a health complaint needs to improve their overall functioning in any way that won't be harmful over the long term. Vitamin therapy can be an amazingly effective adjunct to dietary reform and detoxification.

Some of the earlier natural hygienists were opposed to using vitamins. However, these doctors lived in an era when the food supply was better, when mass human degeneration had not proceeded as far as it has today. From their perspective, it was possible to obtain all the nutrition one needed from food. In our time this is unlikely unless a person knowingly and intelligently produces virtually all their own food on a highly fertile soil body whose fertility is maintained and adjusted with a conscious intent to maximize the nutritive content of the food. Unfortunately, ignorance of the degraded nature of industrial food seems to extend to otherwise admirable natural healing methods such as Macrobiotics and homeopathy because these disciplines also downplay any need for food supplementation.

Vitamins *for* Young Persons *&* Children

Young healthy people from weaning through their thirties should also take nutritional supplements even though young people usually feel so good that they find it impossible to conceive that anything could harm them or that they ever could become seriously sick or actually die. I know this is true because I remember my own youth and besides, why else would young people so glibly ride motorcycles or, after only a few months of brainwashing, charge up a hill into the barrel of a machine gun. Or have unsafe sex in this age of multiple venereal diseases. Until they get a little sense, vitamin supplements help to counteract their inevitable and unpreventable use of recreational foods. Vitamins are the cheapest long life and health insurance plan now available. Parents are generally very surprised at the thought that even their children need nutritional supplements; very few healthy children receive them. A few are given extra vitamin C when acutely ill, when they have colds or communicable diseases such as chicken pox.

Young people require a low dose supplement compared to those of us middle-aged or older, but it should be a broad formula with the full range of vitamins and minerals. Some of the best products I have found over 25 years of research and experimentation with young people are Douglas Cooper's "Basic Formula" (low dose and excellent for children) and "Super T Formula" (double the dose of Basic Formula, therefore better for adolescents and young adults), also from Douglas Cooper Company; Bronson's "Vitamin and Mineral Formula for Active Men and Women" and Bronson's "Insurance Formula." "Vitamin 75 Plus;" and "Formula 2" from Now Natural Foods are also good and less costly.

Healthy very small children who will swallow pills can take these same products at half the recommended dose. If they won't swallow pills the pills can be blended into a fruit smoothie or finely crushed and then stirred into apple sauce. There are also "Children's Chewable Multi-Vitamins + Iron" (1-5 years old) from Douglas Cooper that contains no minerals except iron, Bronson's "Chewable Vitamins" (make sure it is the one for small children, Bronson makes several types of chewables) and a liquid vitamin product from Bronson called Multivitamin Drops for Infants. These will be a little more costly than cutting pills in half.

There is also an extraordinarily high quality multivitamin/mineral formula for children called "Children's Formula Life Extension Mix" from Prolongevity, Ltd. (the Life Extension Foundation), it is in tablet form, and slightly more expensive.

I hope that my book will be around for several generations. The businesses whose vitamin products I recommend will not likely exist in twenty years. Even sooner than that the product names and details of the formulations will almost certainly be altered. So, for future readers discovering this book in a library or dusty shelve of a used book store, if I, at my current level of understanding, were manufacturing a childrens and young adults vitamin formula myself, this is what it would contain. Any commercial formulation within 25 percent of these figures plus or minus would probably be fine as long as the vitamins in the pills were of high quality.

Vitamin C	500 mg	B-1	30 mg
Vitamin E	50 iu	B-2	30 mg
Vitamin A	500 iu	B-3 niacinamide	100 mg
Vitamin D	25 iu	B-5	50 mg
Magnesium	100 mg	B-6	30 mg
Calcium	400 mg	B-12	30 mcg
Selenium	10 mcg	Chromium	20 mcg
Manganese	2 mcg	Biotin	30 mg
Zinc	5 mg	Iodine (as kelp)	5 mg
PABA	20 mg	Bioflavinoids	100 mg

Vitamins *for an* Older Healthy Person

Someone who is beyond 35 to 40 years of age should still feel good almost all of the time. That is how life should be. But enjoying well-being does not mean that no dietary supplementation is called for. The onset of middle age is the appropriate time to begin working on continuing to feel well for as long as possible. Just like a car, if you take very good care of it from the beginning, it is likely to run smoothly for many years into the future. If on the other hand you drive it hard and fast with a lot of deferred maintenance you will probably have to trade it in on a new one after a very few years. Most people in their 70s and older who are struggling with many uncomfortable symptoms and low energy lament, 'if I'd only known I was going to live so long I would have taken better care of myself.' But at that point it is too late for the old donkey; time for a trade in.

Gerontologists refer to combating the aging process as "squaring the curve." We arrive at the peak of our physical function at about age eighteen. How high that peak level is depends on a person's genetic endowment, the quality of the start they received through their mother's nutritional reserves, and the quality of their childhood nutrition and life experience. From that peak our function begins to drop. The rate of drop is not uniform, but is a cascade where each bit of deterioration creates more deterioration, accelerating the rate of deterioration. If various aging experiences were graphed, they would make curves like those on the chart on this page.

Because deterioration starts out so slowly, people usually do not begin to notice there has been any decline until they reach their late 30s. A few fortunate ones don't notice it until their 40s. A few (usually) dishonest ones claim no losses into their 50s but they are almost inevitably lying, either to you or to themselves, or both. Though it might be wisest to begin combating the aging process at age 19, practically speaking, no one is going to start spending substantial money on food supplements until they actually notice significant lost function. For non-athletes this point usually comes when function has dropped to about 90 percent of what it was in our youth. If they're lucky what people usually notice with the beginnings of middle age is an increasing inability for their bodies to tolerate insults such as a night on the town or a big meal. Or they may begin to get colds that just won't seem to go away. Or they may begin coming home after work so tired that they can hardly stay awake and begin falling asleep in their Lazy Boy recliner in front of the TV even before prime time. If they're not so lucky they'll begin suffering the initial twinges of a non-life-threatening chronic condition like arthritis.

The thinnest line demonstrates the worst possible life from a purely physical point of view, where a person started out life with significantly lowered function, lost quite a bit more and then hung on to life for many years without the mercy of death.

If one can postpone the deterioration of aging, they extend and hopefully square the curve (retard loss of function until later and then have the loss occur more rapidly). Someone whose lifetime function resembled a "square curve"(the thickest, topmost line) would experience little or no deterioration until the very end and then would lose function precipitously. At this point we do not know how to eliminate the deterioration but we do know how to slow it down, living longer and feeling better, at least to a point close to the very end.

Vitamin supplements can actually slow or even to a degree, reverse, the aging process. However, to accomplish that task, they have to be taken in amounts far greater than so-called minimum daily requirements, using vitamins as though they were drugs, a therapeutic approach to changing body chemistry profiles and making them resemble a younger body. For example, research gerontologists like Walford reason that if pantothenic acid (vitamin B5), in fairly substantial (but quite safe) doses can extend the life and improve the function of old rats, there is every indication that it will do a similar job on humans. Medical researchers and research gerontologists have noticed that many other vitamin and vitamin-like substances have similar effects on laboratory animals.

Some will object that what helps rats and mice is in no way proven to cause the same result on humans. I agree. Proven with full scientific rigor, no. In fact, at present, the contention is unprovable. Demonstrable as having a high likelihood's of being so, yes! So likely so as to be almost incontrovertible, yes! But provable to the most open-minded, scientific sort–probably not for a long time. However, the Life Extension Foundation is working hard to find some quantifiable method of gauging the aging process in humans without waiting for the inarguable indicator, death. Once this is accomplished and solidly recognized, probably no rational person will be able to doubt that human life span can be increased.

Experiments work far better with short-lived laboratory animals for another reason; we can not control the food and supplement intakes of humans as we can with caged mice. In fact, there are special types of laboratory mice that have been bred to have uniformly short life spans, especially to accelerate this kind of research. With mice we can state accurately that compared to a control group, feeding such and such a dose of such and such a supplement extended the life-span or functional performance by such and such a percent.

A lot of these very same medical gerontologists nourish their own bodies as thoroughly as the laboratory animals they are studying, taking broad mixes of food supplements at doses proportional to those that extend the life spans of their research animals. This approach to using supplementation is at the other end of the scale compared to using supplements to prevent gross deficiencies. In the life extension approach, vitamins and vitamin-like substances are used as a therapy against the aging process itself.

Will it work? Well, some of these human guinea pigs have been on heavy vitamin supplementation for over thirty years (as of 1995) and none seem to be suffering any damage. Will they live longer? It is impossible to say with full scientific rigor? To know if life extension works, we would have to first determine "live longer than what?" After all, we don't know how long any person might have lived without life extending vitamin supplements. Though it can't be "proven," it makes perfect sense to me to spend far less money on an intensive life extension vitamin program than I would certainly lose as a result of age-related sickness.

Besides, I've already observed from personal use and from results in my clinical practice that life extension vitamin programs do work. Whether I and my clients will ultimately live longer or not, the people who I have put on these programs, including myself and my husband, usually report that for several years after starting they find themselves feeling progressively younger, gradually returning to an overall state of greater well-being they knew five or ten or fifteen years ago. They have more energy, feel clearer mentally, have fewer unwanted somatic symptoms.

Sometimes the improvements seem rather miraculous. After a few months on the program one ninety year old man, an independent-minded Oregonian farmer, reported that he began awakening with an erection every morning; unfortunately, his 89 year old cranky and somewhat estranged wife, who would not take vitamins, did not appreciate this youthfulness. A few months later (he had a small farm) he planted a holly orchard. Most of you won't appreciate what this means without a bit of explanation, but in Oregon, holly is grown as a high-priced and highly profitable ornamental for the clusters of leaves and berries. But a slow-growing holly orchard takes 25 years to began making a profit!

A few older clients of mine reported that they noticed nothing from the life extension program, but these are unique people who have developed the ability to dominate their bodies with their minds and routinely pay their bodies absolutely no attention, driving them relentlessly to do their will. Usually they use their energies to accomplish good, Christian works. Eventually, these dedicated and high-toned people break down and die like everyone else. Will they do so later on life extending vitamins than they would have otherwise? I couldn't know because I can't know how long they might have lived without supplementation and since they refuse to admit the vitamins do them any good, they won't pay for them.

Many on life extension programs experience a reverse aging process for awhile. However, after the full benefit of the supplementation has worked itself through their body chemistry, they again begin to experience the aging process. I believe the process will then be slowed by their vitamins compared to what it would have been without supplements. But I can't prove it. Maybe we will have some idea if the program worked 20 to 40 years from now.

At this time I know of only two companies that make top quality life extension vitamin supplement formulas. One is Prolongevity (Life Extension Foundation), the other, Vitamin Research Products. I prefer to support what I view as the altruistic motives behind Prolongevity and buy my products from them. Unfortunately, these vitamin compounders can not put every possibly beneficial substance in a single bottle of tablets. The main reason they do not is fear of the power-grabbing Food and Drug Administration. This agency is threatening constantly to remove certain of the most useful life-extending substances from the vitamin trade and make them the exclusive property of prescription-writing medical doctors. So far, public pressure has been mobilized against the FDA every time action was threatened and has not permitted this. If some product were included in a mix and that product were prohibited, the entire mixed, bottled and labeled batch that remained unsold at that time would be wasted, at enormous cost.

Were I manufacturing my own life extension supplement I would include the following. By the way, to get this all in one day, it is necessary to take 6 to 12 large tablets daily, usually spread throughout the day, taken a few at a time with each meal. If you compare my suggested formulation to another one, keep in mind that variations of 25 percent one way or another won't make a significant difference, and adding other beneficial substances to my recommendations probably is only helpful. However, I would not want to eliminate anything in the list below, it is the minimum:

Beta-Carotene	25,000 iu	Selenium	100 mcg
Vitamin A	5,000 iu	Taurine	500 mg
B-1	250 mg	Cyctine	200 mg
B-2	50 mg	Gluthaianone	15 mg
B-3 niacinamid	850 mg	Choline	650 mg
B-5	750 mg	Inositol	250 mg
B-6	200 mg	Flavanoids	500 mg
B-12	100 mcg	Zinc	35 mg
PABA	50 mg	Chromium	100 mcg
Folic Acid	500 mcg	Molybdenum	123 mg
Biotin	200 mcg	Manganese	5 mg
Vitamin C	3,000mg	Iodine (as kelp)	10 mg
Vitamin E	600 iu	Co-Enzyme Q-10	60 mg
Magnesium	1,000 mg	DMAE	100 mg
Potassium	100 mg	Ginko biloba	120 mg
Calcium	1,000 mg	Vitamin D-3	200 iu

Please also keep in mind that there are many other useful substances not listed above. For example, every day I have a "green drink," an herbal preparation containing numerous tonic substances like ginseng and also various forms of algae and chlorophyll extracts. My green drink makes my body feel very peppy all day, so it certainly enhances my life and may extend it. It costs about $25,00 a month to enjoy that. I also use various pure amino acids at times. Phenylalyanine will make me get more aggressive whenever I am feeling a little lackluster; this nutrient has also been used as an effective therapy against depression. Melatonin taken at bedtime really does help me get to sleep and may have remarkable life-extending properties. Other amino acids help my body manufacture growth hormones and I use them from the time I begin training seriously in spring through the end of the summer triathlon competition season. Pearson and Shaw's book (see Bibliography) is a good starting point to begin learning about this remarkably useful subject.

The Future *of* Life Extension

I beg the readers indulgence for a bit of futurology about what things may look like if the life extension movement continues to develop.

Right now, a full vitamin and vitamin-like substance life extension program costs between $50 and $100 dollars per month. However, pharmaceutical researchers occasionally notice that drugs meant to treat and cure diseases, when tested on lab animals for safety, make these animals live quite a bit longer and function better. Though the FDA doesn't allow any word of this to be printed in official prescribing data, the word does get around to other researchers, to gerontologists and eventually to that part of the public that is eagerly looking for longer life. Today there are numerous people who routinely take prescription medicines meant to cure a disease they do not have and plan to take those medicines for the rest of their long, long life.

These drugs being patented, the tariff gets a lot steeper compared to taking vitamins. (Since they are naturally-occurring substances, vitamins can't be patented and therefore, aren't big-profit items. Perhaps that's one reason the FDA is so covertly opposed to vitamins.) Right now it would be quite possible to spend many hundred dollars per month on a life extension program that included most of these potentially beneficent prescription drugs.

As more of life-extending substances are discovered, the cost of participating in a maximally effective life extension program will escalate. However, those who can afford chemically enhanced functioning will enjoy certain side-benefits. Their productive, enjoyable life spans may measure well over a century, perhaps approaching two centuries or more. Some of these substances greatly improve intelligence so they will become brighter and have faster reaction times. With more time to accumulate more wisdom and experience than "short livers" these folks will become wiser, too. They will have more time to compound their investment assets and thus will become far more wealthy. They will become an obvious and recognizable aristocracy. This new upper class will immediately recognize each other on the street because they will look entirely different than the short-lived poorer folk and will probably run the political economic system.

And this new aristocratic society I see coming may be far more pleasant than the one dominated by the oligarchy we now have covertly running things. For with greater age and experience does really come greater wisdom. I have long felt that the biggest problem with Earth is that we did not live long enough. As George Bernard Shaw quipped when he was 90 (he lived to 96), "here I am, 90 years old, just getting out of my adolescence and getting some sense, and my body is falling apart as fast as it can."

Vitamin Program For The Sick

No matter which way you look at it or how well insured you may be against it, being sick is expensive (not to mention what it does to one's quality of life), and by far the best thing to do is to prevent it from happening in the first place. However, most people do not do anything about their health until forced to by some painful condition. If you are already sick there are a number of supplements you can take which have the potential to shorten the duration and severity of the illness, and hopefully prevent a recurrence.

The sicker you are, the more supplements you will require; as health is regained, the dosage and variety of substances can be reduced. In chronic illness, megadoses of many nutrients are usually beneficial. Any sick adult should begin a life extension vitamin program unless they are highly allergic to so many things already that they can not tolerate many kinds of vitamins as well. In addition to the life extension program, vitamin C should be taken by the chronically ill at a dose from 10 to 25 grams daily, depending on the severity of the condition.

Many people want to know whether or not they should take their regular food supplements during a fast. On a water fast most supplements in a hard tablet form will not be broken down at all, and often can be seen floating by in the colonic viewing tube looking exactly like it did when you swallowed it. This waste can be avoided by crushing or chewing (yuck) the tablets, before swallowing. Encapsulated vitamins usually are absorbed, but if you want to make sure, open the capsule and dump it in the back of your mouth before swallowing with water. Powdered vitamins are well absorbed.

On a water fast the body is much more sensitive to any substance introduced, so as a general rule it is not a good idea to take more than one half your regular dose of food supplements. Most fasters do fine without any supplements. Many people get an upset stomach from supplements on an empty stomach, and these people should not take any during a water fast unless they develop symptoms of mineral deficiencies (usually a pre-existing condition) such as leg cramps and tremors, these symptoms necessitate powdered or well-chewed-up mineral supplement. Minerals don't taste too bad to chew, just chalky.

The same suggestions regarding dosage of supplements for a water fast are also true for a juice fast or vegetable broth fast. On a raw food cleansing diet the full dose of supplements should be taken with meals.

There exists an enormous body of data about vitamins; books and magazine articles are always touting some new product or explaining the uses of an old one. If you want to know more about using ordinary vitamins you'll find leads in the bibliography to guide your reading. However, there is one "old" vitamin and a few newer and relatively unknown life extending substances that are so useful and important to handling illness that I would like to tell you more about them.

Vitamin C is not a newly discovered vitamin, but was one of the first ever identified. If you are one of those people that just hate taking vitamins, and you were for some reason willing to take only one, vitamin C would be your best choice. Vitamin C would be the clear winner because it helps enormously with any infection and in invaluable in tissue healing and rebuilding collagen. If I was going on a long trip and didn't want to pack a lot of weight, my first choice would be to insure three to six grams of vitamin C for daily use when I was healthy (I'd take the optimum dose–ten grams a day–if weight were no limitation). I'd also carry enough extra C to really beef up my intake when dealing with an unexpected acute illness or accident.

When traveling to faraway places, exposed to a whole new batch of organisms, frequently having difficulty finding healthy foods, going through time zones, losing nights of sleep, it is easy to become enervated enough to catch a local cold or flu. If I have brought lots of extra vitamin C with me I know that my immune system will be able to conquer just about anything–as long as I also stop eating and can take an enema. I also like to have vitamin C as a part of my first aid kit because if I experience a laceration, a sprain, broken bone, or a burn, I can increase my internal intake as well as apply it liberally directly on the damaged skin surface. Vitamin C can be put directly in the eye in a dilute solution with distilled water for infections and injuries, in the ear for ear infections, and in the nose for sinus infections. If you are using the acid form of C (ascorbic acid) and it smarts too much, make a more dilute solution, or switch to the alkaline form of C (calcium ascorbate) which can be used as a much more concentrated solution without a stinging sensation. Applied directly on the skin C in solution makes a very effective substitute for sun screen. It doesn't filter out ultraviolet, it beefs up the skin to better deal with the insult.

I believe vitamin C can deal with a raging infection such as pneumonia as well or better than antibiotics. But to do that, C is going to have to be administered at the maximum dose the body can process. This is easily discoverable by a 'bowel tolerance test' which basically means you keep taking two or three grams of C each hour, (preferably in the powdered, most rapidly assimilable form) until you get a runny stool (the trots). The loose stool happens when there is so much C entering the small intestine that it is not all absorbed, but is instead, passed through to the large intestine. At that point cut back just enough that the stool is only a little loose, not runny. At this dose, your blood stream will be as saturated by vitamin C as you can achieve by oral ingestion.

It can make an important difference which type of vitamin C is taken because many people are unable to tolerate the acid form of C beyond 8 or 10 grams a day, but they can achieve a therapeutic dose without discomfort with the alkaline (buffered) vitamin C products such as calcium ascorbate, sodium ascorbate, or magnesium-potassium ascorbates.

Vitamin C also speeds up the healing of internal tissues and damaged connective tissue. Damaged internal tissues might include stomach ulcers (use the alkaline form of vitamin C only), bladder and kidney infections (acid form usually best), arthritic disorders with damage to joints and connective tissue (alkaline form usually best). Sports injuries heal up a lot faster with a therapeutic dose of vitamin C. As medicine, vitamin C should be taken at the rate of one or two grams every two hours (depending on the severity of the condition), spaced out to avoid unnecessary losses in the urine which happens if it were taken ten grams at a time. If you regularly use the acid form of vitamin C powder, which is the cheapest, be sure to use a straw and dissolve it in water or juice so that the acid does not dissolve the enamel on your teeth over time.

And this is as good a point as any to mention that just like broccoli is not broccoli, a vitamin is not necessarily a vitamin. Vitamins are made by chemical and pharmaceutical companies. To make this confusion even more interesting, the business names that appear on vitamin bottles are not the real manufacturers. Bronson's Pharmaceuticals is a distributor and marketer, not a manufacturer. The same is true of every vitamin company I know of. These companies buy bulk product by the barrel or sack; then encapsulate, blend and roll pills, bottle and label, advertise and make profit. The point of all this is that some actual vitamin manufacturers produce very high quality products and others shortcut. Vitamin distributors must make ethical (or unethical) choices about their suppliers.

It is beyond the scope of this book to be a manual for going into the vitamin business. However, there are big differences in how effective vitamins with the same chemical name are and the differences hinge on who actually brewed them up.

For example, there are at least two quality levels of vitamin C on the market right now. The pharmaceutical grade is made by Roche or BASF. Another form, it could be called "the bargain barrel brew," is made in China. Top quality vitamin C is quite a bit more costly; as I write this, the price differential is about 40 percent between the cheap stuff and the best. This can make a big difference in bottle price and profit. Most of the discount retail vitamin companies use the Chinese product.

There's more than a price difference. The vitamin C from China contains measurable levels of lead, cadmium, mercury, iron and other toxic metals. The FDA allows this slightly contaminated product to be sold in the US because the Recommended Daily Allowance for vitamin C is a mere 60 milligrams per day. Taken at that level, the toxic metals would, as the FDA sees it, do no harm. However, many users of vitamin C take 100–200 times the RDA. The cheap form of C would expose them to potentially toxic levels of heavy metal poisons. The highly refined top-quality product removes impurities to a virtually undetectable level.

I buy my C from Bronson who ethically gives me the quality stuff. I know for a fact that the vitamin C sold by Prolongevity is also top quality. I've had clients who bought cheaper C than Bronson's and discovered it was not quite like Bronson's in appearance or taste. More importantly, it did not seem to have the same therapeutic effect.

The distributors I've mentioned so far, Bronson, NOW, Cooper, Prolongevity and Vitamin Research Products are all knowledgeable about differences between actual manufacturers and are ethical, buying and reselling only high quality products. Other distributors I believe to be reputable include Twin Labs, Schiff and Plus. I know there are many other distributors with high ethic levels but I can not evaluate all their product lines. And as I've mentioned earlier, businesses come and go rather quickly, but I hope my book will be read for decades. I do know that I would be very reluctant to buy my vitamins at a discount department store or supermarket; when experimenting with new suppliers I have at times been severely disappointed.

Co-enzyme Q-10. This substance is normally manufactured in the human body and is also found in minuscule amounts in almost every cell on Earth. For that reason it is also called "ubiquinone." But this vitamin has been only recently discovered, so as I write this book Co-enzyme Q-10 is not widely known.

Q-10 is essential to the functioning of the mitochondria, that part of the cell that produces energy. With less Q-10 in heart cells, for example, the heart has less energy and pumps less. The same is true of the immune system cells, the liver cells, every cell. As we age the body is able to make less and less Q-10, contributing to the loss of energy frequently experienced with age, as well as the diminished effectiveness of the immune system, and a shortened life span.

Q-10 was first used for its ability to revitalize heart cells. It was a prescription medicine in Japan. But unlike other drugs used to stimulate the heart, at any reasonable dose Q-10 has no harmful side effects. It also tends to give people the extra pick up they are trying to get out of a cup of coffee. But Q-10 does so by improving the function of every cell in the body, not by whipping exhausted adrenals like caffeine does. Q-10 is becoming very popular with athletes who measure their overall cellular output against known standards.

Besides acting as a general tonic, when fed to lab animals, Co-Enzyme Q-10 makes them live 33 to 45 percent longer!

DMAE is another extremely valuable vitamin-like substance that is not widely known. It is a basic building material that the body uses to make acetylcholine, the most generalized neurotransmitter in the body. Small quantities of DMAE are found in fish, but the body usually makes it in a multi-stage synthesis that starts with the amino acid choline, arrives at DMAE at about step number three and ends up finally with acetylcholine.

The body's nerves are wrapped in fatty tissue that should be saturated with acetylcholine. Every time a nerve impulse is transmitted from one nerve cell to the next, a molecule of acetylcholine is consumed. Thus acetylcholine has to be constantly replaced. As the body ages, levels of acetylcholine surrounding the nerves drop and in consequence, the nerves begin to deteriorate. DMAE is rapidly and easily converted into acetylcholine and helps maintain acetylcholine levels in older people at a youthful level.

When laboratory rats are fed DMAE they solve mazes more rapidly, remember better, live about 40 percent longer than rats not fed DMAE and most interestingly, when autopsied, their nervous systems resemble those of a young rat, without any evidence of the usual deterioration of aging. Human nervous systems also deteriorate with age, especially those of people suffering from senility. It is highly probable that DMAE will do the same thing to us. DMAE also smoothes out mood swings in humans and seems to help my husband, Steve, when he has a big writing project. He can keep working without getting 'writers block', fogged out, or rollercoastering.

DMAE is a little hard to find. Prolongevity and VRP sell it in powder form. Since the FDA doesn't know any MDR and since the product is not capped up, the bottle of powder sagely states that one-quarter teaspoonful contains 333 milligrams. Get the hint? DMAE tastes a little like sour salt and one-quarter teaspoonful dissolves readily in water every morning before breakfast, or anytime for that matter. DMAE is also very inexpensive considering what it does. A year's supply costs about $20.

Lecithin is a highly tonic and inexpensive food supplement that is underutilized by many people even though it is easily obtainable in healthfood stores. It is an emulsifier, breaking fats down into small separate particles, keeping blood cholesterol emulsified to prevent arterial deposits. Taken persistently, lecithin partially and slowly eliminates existing cholesterol deposits from the circulatory system.

In our cholesterol-frightened society lecithin should be a far more popular supplement than it currently is. It is easy to take either as a food in the granular form or when encapsulated. Lecithin granules have very little flavor and can be added to a home-made vinegar and oil salad dressing, where they emulsify the oil and make it blend with the vinegar, thickening the mixture and causing it to stick to the salad better. Lecithin can also be put in a fruits smoothie. A scant tablespoon a day is sufficient. Try to buy the kind of lecithin that has the highest phosphatidyl choline content because this substance is the second benefit of taking lecithin. Phosphatidyl choline is another precursor used by the body to build acetylcholine and helps maintain the nervous system.

Algae. Spirulina or sun dried chlorella are also great food supplements. Both make many people feel energized, pepped-up. It is possible to fast on either product and still maintain sufficient energy levels to take of minimal work responsibilities. Algae reduces appetite and as a dietary supplement can assist in weight loss. It contains large amounts of highly-assimilable protein due to it's high chlorophyll content, as well as a large amount of beta carotene. It also assists in detoxification of the lymphatic system. It can be purchased as tablets or powder. Take a heaping teaspoon daily, or at least six tablets.

Chapter Seven

The Analysis *of* Disease States: Helping *the* Body Recover

From the Hygienic Dictionary

Diagnosis. [1] In the United States, making a diagnosis implies that you are a doctor duly licensed to engage in diagnostic function.... The making of a diagnosis is reserved only for doctors.... The term "analysis" does not have such an explicit legal definition. Thus, it is the term of choice of iridologists and the one most often used by them. It is essential for the survival and promotion of iridology that those who choose to engage in its practice avoid naming any disease condition. As we have seen, to do so is to infringe on rights reserved exclusively for doctors and can land the iridologist, sooner or later, in a snarl of legal troubles.

It is better for the iridologist to refrain from suggesting to a person that he has any particular disease, letting such diagnostics remain the province of licensed doctors. In so doing, the iridologist will avoid transgressing the law and stepping on the toes of those who are legally qualified to diagnose.

It is indeed unfortunate that one of the greatest pitfalls awaiting the iridologist is the temptation to name diseases. The feelings of satisfaction and power resulting from conferring a name are deeply rooted in the human psyche. For example, the Bible tells us that man's first task on Earth was to name the animals, thus giving him power and dominion over them.

Strong is the temptation to name diseases because nearly everyone has come to expect that his malady has a name. Patients have come to expect, and doctors have been trained to make, a diagnosis. . . . "After all," the patient may reason, "how can you hope to deal with my condition if you aren't knowledgeable enough to call it by name?"

It is not necessary to name diseases in order to exercise dominion over them.

Dr. Bernard Jensen, Visions of Health.

In self defense, I must make it very clear from the first word that hygienists and most other naturopaths of various persuasions, and especially I myself, have never in the past, never!, and do not now, diagnose, treat or offer to cure, disease or illness. Diagnosis and curing are sole, exclusive privileges of certified, duly-licensed medical doctors and may only be done with a grant of Authority to do so from the State. Should an unlicensed person diagnose, offer to treat or attempt to cure disease or illness, they will have committed a felonious act. With big penalties. Therefore, I do not do it.

When one of my clients comes to me and says that a medical doctor says they have some disease or other, I agree that the medical doctor says they have some disease or other, and I never dare say that they don't. Or even confirm on my own authority that I think they do have some disease or other.

What I can legally do for a client is to analyze the state of their body and its organs, looking for weaknesses and apparent allergies. I can lawfully state that I think their liver tests weak, the pancreas appears not to be functioning well in terms of handling meat digestion, that the kidney is having a hard time of it. I can say I see a lump sticking out of their body when one is obviously sticking out of their body; I can not say that lump is cancerous but I can state that the cells in that lump test overly strong and that if I myself had a mass of growing cells testing overly strong and if I believed in the standard medical model, then I would be rushing my overly strong testing cells to an oncologist. But I don't dare say the person has a cancer. Or diabetes. Or is getting close to kidney failure. That is a diagnosis.

To me, diagnosis is a form of magic rite in which the physician discovers the secret name of the devil that is inhabiting one's body and then, knowing that secret name, performs the correct rite and ritual to cast that demon out. I don't know why people are made so happy knowing the name of their condition! Does it really matter? Either the body can heal the condition or it can't. If it can, you will recover (especially if you give the body a little help). If the body can't heal a condition you will die or live a long time being miserable. No "scientific" medical magic can do better than that.

By describing a disease in terms of its related organ weaknesses, instead of pinning a Latin name on it, I am able to assist the body to achieve recovery in a superior way that the physician rarely does. By discovering that the body with the lump of overly strong cells also has a weak spleen, liver and thymus gland, I can take actions to strengthen the spleen, liver and thymus. If the body can strengthen its spleen, liver and thymus, then the overly strong cells miraculously vanish. But of course I and what I did did not cure any disease. Any improvements that happen I assign (correctly) to the body's own healing power.

The way I analyze the organic integrity of the body is through a number of related methods, including the general appearance of the body, the patient's health history, various clues such as body and breath odor, skin color and tone, and especially, biokinesiology, the applied science of muscle testing. Biokinesiology can be used to test the strength or weakness of specific organs and their function. A weak latissimus dorsi muscle indicates a weak pancreas, for example. Specific acupuncture points can be tested in conjunction with muscle strength to indicate the condition of specific organs or glands. The strength of the arm's resistance to downward pressure could be calibrated with a spring scale and precisely gauged, but experienced practitioners have no need for this bother, because they are able to pick up subtle changes in the arms resistance that are not apparent to the testee. Thus muscle testing becomes an art form, and becomes as effective as the person using it is sensitive and aware.

Biokinesiology works because every organ and gland in the body is interconnected with other parts of the body through nerve pathways and nerve transmissions, which are electrical and can be measured through muscle testing. This may seem too esoteric for the "scientific" among you, but acupuncture points and energy manifestations around and in the body—are now accepted phenomena, their reality demonstrated by special kinds of photography. Acupuncturists, who heal by manipulating the body's energy field with metal needles, are now widely accepted in the western hemisphere. Kinesiology utilizes the same acupuncture points (and some others too) for analytic purposes so it is sometimes called "contact reflex analysis."

I have studied and used Kinesiology for 25 years with the majority of my clients with very good success. There are some few people who are very difficult to test because they are either too debilitated, lack electrical conductivity, or their state of mind is so skeptical and negative about this type of approach that they put up an impenetrable mental barrier and/or hold their body so rigidly that I can hardly determine a response. A skilled can overcome the obstacle of a weak body that can barely respond, but the person who is mentally opposed and determined to prove you wrong should not be tested. If you proceed it is sure to have an unsatisfactory outcome for all concerned. For even if I manage to accurately analyze the condition of a skeptical client, they will never believe the analysis and will not follow suggestions.

The "scientific," open-minded, "reasonable" client can be better approached using an academic-like discussion based on published literature that demonstrates how people with similar symptoms and complaints do very well on a particular dietary regimen and supplements. This type of person will sometimes follow dietary recommendations to the last letter, because their scientific background has trained them to be obedient.

When a client comes to me, I like to take a real good look at who is sitting in front of me. I take my leisure to find out all about their history, their complaints, their motivation to change, their experience with natural healing, their level of personal responsibility, whether or not they have to work, whether or not they can take time out to heal, will they fast or take supplements, do they have sufficient finances to carry a program through to a successful completion, do they have people closely connected to them that are strongly opposed to alternative approaches, can they withstand some discomfort and self-denial, do they have toxic relationships with other people that are contributing to their condition, are they willing to read and educate themselves in greater depth about natural healing, etc. I need to know the answers to these questions in order to help them choose a program which is most likely to succeed.

Even though fasting is the most effective method I know of, it is not for people who are compelled to keep up a work schedule, nor is it for people who are very ill and do not have anyone to assist them and supervise them. Nor is it for people who do not understand fasting and are afraid of it. People who have associates that are opposed to it, and people who do not have a strongly-functioning liver or kidneys should not fast either. Seriously ill people that have been on a meat-heavy diet with lots of addicting substances need a long runway into a fast so as to not overwhelm their organs of elimination. Does the person in front of me have an eating disorder, or an otherwise suicidal approach to fasting, etc. Clearly fasting is not for everyone, and if I recommend it to the wrong person, the result will be a bad reputation for a marvelous tool.

Given that many clients can not fast without a lot of preparation, the majority of my clients start out with a gentle detox program that takes considerably more time, but works. These gradients have been outlined under the healing programs for the chronically ill, acutely ill, etc.

To help rebuild poorly functioning organs, I sometimes use a specialized group of food supplements called protomorphogens. These are not readily available to the general public and perhaps should not be casually purchasable like vitamins, because, as with many prescription drugs, supervision is usually necessary for their successful use. If the FDA ever succeeds at making protomorphogens unavailable to me, I could still have very good results. (At this time the Canadian authorities do not allow importation of protomorphogens for resale, though individuals can usually clear small shipments through Canada Customs if for their own personal use.) But protomorphogens do facilitate healing and sometimes permit healing to occur at a lower gradient of handling. Without them a body might have to fast to heal, with the aid of protomorphogens a person might be able to get better without fasting. And if protomorphogens are used (chewed up–ugh!) while fasting, healing is accelerated.

Protomorphogens are made from freeze-dried, organically-raised animal organ meats (usually calf or lamb) combined with very specific vitamins, herbs and other co-factors to potentiate the effect. I view protomorphogens as containing nutritional supplementation specific for the rebuilding of the damaged organ.

Doctor Royal Lee, a medical genius who developed protomorphogens therapy in the 50s and who spent several stints in prison in exchange for his benevolence and concern for human well-being, also founded the company that has supplied me with protomorphogens. After decades of official persecution and denial of the efficacy of protomorphogens by the power structure, it looks like they are about to finally have their day. As I write this book cutting-edge medical research companies are developing therapies using concentrated animal proteins (protomorphogens) to treat arthritis, multiple sclerosis, eye inflamations and juvenile diabetes. The researchers talk as though they are highly praiseworthy for "discovering" this approach.

Unfortunately, this development is likely to cut two ways. On one hand, it vindicates Dr. Lee; on the other, when these drug companies find a way to patent their materials, they may finally succeed at forcing protomorphogens (currently quite inexpensive) off the non-prescription market and into the restricted and profitable province of the MD.

I divide clients into two basic types: simple cases and complex ones. When I was treating mental illness, occasionally I had a client who had not been sick for too long. I could usually make this client well quite easily. But if the person had already become institutionalized, had been psychotic for many years, had received much prior treatment, then their case had been made much more difficult. This sort had a poor prognosis. A very similar situation exists with physical illnesses. Many people get sick only because they lack information about how to keep themselves healthy and about what made them sick. Once they find out the truth, they take my medicine without complaint and almost inevitably get better very rapidly. Some of these people can be quite ill when they first come to me but usually they have not been sick for very long. Their intention when coming into my office is very positive and have no counter intentions to getting better. There are no spiritual or psychological reasons that they deserve to be sick. If this person had not found me, they almost certainly would have found some other practitioner who would have made them well. This type of person honestly feels they are entitled to wellness. And they are.

However, some of the sick are not sick for lack of life-style information; they suffer from a mental/spiritual malady as well, one that inevitably preceded their illness by many years. In fact, their physical ailments are merely reflections of underlying problems. This patient's life is usually a snarl of upsets, problems, and guilty secrets. Their key relationships are usually vicious or unhealthy. Their level of interpersonal honesty may be poor. There are usually many things about their lives they do not confront and so, can not change. With this type of case, all the physical healing in the world will not make them permanently better because the mental and emotional stresses they live under serve as a constant source of enervation.

Cases like this usually do not have only one thing wrong with them. They almost always have been sick for a long time; most have been what I call "doctor hoppers," confused by contrary diagnoses and conflicting MD opinions. When I get a case like this I know from the first that healing is going to be a long process, and a dubious one at that. On the physical level, their body will only repair one aspect of their multiple illnesses at a time. Simultaneously, they must be urged to confront their life on a gentle gradient. There is usually a lot of backsliding and rollercoastering. The detoxification process, physical and psychological, can take several years and must happen on all the levels of their life. This kind of case sees only gradual improvement interspersed with periods of worsening that indicate there remains yet another level of mental unawareness that has to be unraveled.

Few medical doctors or holistic therapists really understand or can help this kind of case. To do so, the doctor has to be in touch with their own reactive mind and their own negative, evil impulses (which virtually all humans have). Few people, including therapists, are willing to be aware of their own dark side. But when we deny it in ourselves, we must pretend it doesn't exist in others, and become its victim instead of conquering it. Anyone who denies that they have or are influenced by their own darker aspects who seem to be totally sweet and light, is lying; proof of this is that they still are here on Earth.

All this generalizing about diagnostic methods and clinical approaches could go on for chapters and more chapters, and writing them would be fine if I were teaching a group of health clinicians that were reading this book to become better practitioners. But I'm sure most of my readers are far more interested in some complaint of their own or in the health problem of a loved one, and are intensely interested in one might go about handling various conditions and complaints, what types of organ weaknesses are typically associated with them, and what approaches I usually recommend to encourage healing. And, most importantly, what kind of success or lack of it have I had over the past twenty five years, encouraging the healing of various conditions with hygienic methods.

In the case studies that follow I will mostly report the simpler, easier-to-fix problems because that is what most people have; still, many of these involve life-threatening or quality-of-life-destroying illnesses. I will tell the success story of one very complicated, long-suffering case that involved multiple levels of psychological and spiritual handling as well as considerable physical healing.

Arthritis

Some years back my 70 years old mother came from the family homestead in the wilds of northern British Columbia to visit me at the Great Oaks School. She had gotten into pathetic physical condition. Fifteen years previously she had remarried. Tom, her new husband, had been a gold prospector and general mountain man, a wonderfully independent and cantankerous cuss, a great hunter and wood chopper and all around good-natured backwoods homestead handyman. Tom had tired of solitary log cabin life and to solve his problem had taken on the care and feeding of a needy widow, my mom. He began doing the cooking and menu planning. Tom, a little older than my mother, had no sense about eating but could still shoot game. Ever since their marriage she had been living on moose meat stews with potatoes and gravy, white flour bread with jam, black tea with canned milk, a ritual glass of brandy at bedtime, and almost no fresh fruit or vegetables.

In her youth, my mother had been a concert pianist; now she had such large arthritic knobs on all of her knuckles that her hands had become claws. Though there was still that very same fine upright in the cabin that I had learned to play as a child, she had long since given up the piano. Her knees also had large arthritic knobs; this proud woman with a straight back and long, flowing strides was bent over, limping along with a cane. She was also 30 pounds overweight and her blood pressure was a very dangerous 210 over 140, just asking for a stroke.

Instead of a welcoming feast, the usual greeting offered to a loved one who has not been seen for a few years, I immediately started her on a juice fast. I gave her freshly prepared carrot juice (one quart daily) mixed with wheat grass juice (three ounces daily) plus daily colonics. She had no previous experience with these techniques but she gamely accepted everything I threw her way because she knew I was doing it because I loved her and wanted to see her in better condition. She also received a daily full body massage with particular attention to the hand and knees, stimulating the circulation to the area and speeding the removal of wastes. Every night her hands and knees were wrapped in warm castor oil compresses held in place with old sheeting.

I did not use any vitamins or food supplements in her case. I did give her flavorful herbal teas made of peppermint and chamomile because she needed the comfort of a hot cupa; but these teas were in no way medicinal except for her morale.

In three weeks on this program, Grannybelle, as I and my daughters called her, had no unsightly knobs remaining on either her knuckles or knees and she could walk and move her fingers without pain within a normal range of movement. The big payoff for me besides seeing her look so wonderful (20 years younger and 20 pounds lighter) was to hear her sit down and treat us to a Beethoven recital. And her blood pressure was 130 over 90.

Breast Cancer

I have worked with many young women with breast cancer; so many in fact, that their faces and cases tend to blur. But whenever I think about them, Kelly inevitably comes to mind because we became such good friends. Like me, Kelly was an independent-minded back country Canuck. At the age 26, she received a medical diagnosis of breast cancer. Kelly had already permitted a lumpectomy and biopsy, but had studied the statistical outcomes and did not want to treat her illness with radical mastectomy, radiation and chemotherapy because she knew her odds of long-term survival without radical medical treatment were equal to or better than allowing the doctors to do everything possible. Nor did she want to lose even one of her breasts. She knew how useful her breasts were because she had already suckled one child, not to mention their contribution to one's own self-image as a whole person. I admired Kelly's unusual independent-mindedness because she comes from a country where universal health coverage is in place; her insurance would have paid all the costs had she been willing to accept conventional medicine, but Canadian national health insurance does not cover alternative therapy.

Kelly stayed with me for nearly two months as a residential faster, because she needed to be far from the distractions of a troubled family life. With financial support from her parents and child-care from her friends she was able to take time out to give the recovery of health top priority in her life without worrying about whether her small son was being well cared for. This peace of mind was also very important to her recovery.

Analysis with biokinesiology showed a pervasively weak immune system, including a weak thymus gland, spleen, and an overloaded lymphatic system. Her liver was weak, but not as weak as it might have been, because she had become a vegetarian, and had been working on her health in a haphazard fashion for a few years. Kelly's body also showed weaknesses in pancreatic and adrenal function as well as a toxic colon. Most immediately worrisome to her, biokinesiology testing showed several over-strong testing lumpy areas in the breasts and over-strong testing lumpy lymph nodes in the armpits. Cancerous tumors always test overly strong

Kelly's earlier life-style had contributed to her condition in several ways. She had worked for years in a forestry tree nursery handling seedling trees treated with highly toxic chemicals. She had worked as a cook in a logging camp for several seasons, eating too much meat and greasy food. And she had also spent the usual number of adolescent and young adult years deeply involved in recreational drug use and the bad diet that went with it.

Kelly started right in on a rigorous water fast that lasted for one entire month. She had a colonic every day, plus body work including reflexology, holding and massage of neurolymphatic and neurovascular points, and stimulation of acupuncture points related to weak organ systems and general massage to stimulate overall circulation and lymphatic drainage. She took protomorphogens to help rebuild her weakened organs; she took ten grams of vitamin C every day and a half-dose of life extension vitamin mix in assimilable powdered form; she drank herbal teas of echinacea and fenugreek seeds and several ounces of freshly squeezed wheat grass juice every day. Twice each day she made poultices out of clay and the pulp left over from making her wheat grass juice, filled an old bra with this mixture and pressed it to her breast for several hours until the clay dried. Shortly, I will explain all the measures in some detail.

These physical therapies were accompanied by counseling sessions dealing with some severe and long-unresolved problems, response patterns and relationships that triggered her present illness. Her son's father (Kelly's ex) was suppressive and highly intimidating. Fearful of him, Kelly seemed unable to successfully extricate herself from the relationship due to the ongoing contact which revolved over visitation and care of their son. But Kelly had grit! While fasting, she confronted these tough issues in her life and unflinchingly made the necessary decisions. When she returned to Canada she absolutely decided, without any nagging doubts, reservations or qualifications, to make any changes necessary to ensure her survival. Only after having made these hard choices could she heal.

I one respect, Kelly was a highly unusual faster. Throughout the entire month on water, Kelly took daily long walks, frequently stopping to lie down and rest in the sun on the way. She would climb to or from the top of a very large and steep hill nearby. She never missed a day, rain or shine.

At the end of her month on water Kelly's remaining breast lumps had disappeared, the lymphatic system and immune system tested strong, as well as the liver, pancreas, adrenals, and large intestine. No areas tested overly strong.

She broke the fast with the same discipline she had conducted it, on carrot juice, a cup every two hours. After three days on juice she began a raw food diet with small servings of greens and sprouts well chewed, interspersed at two hour intervals with fresh juicy fruits. After about ten days on "rabbit food," she eased into avocados, cooked vegetables, nuts, seeds, and whole grains and then went home.

As I write this, it is eight years since Kelly's long fast. She still comes to see me every few years to check out her diet and just say hello. She has had two more children by a new, and thoroughly wonderful husband and suckled them both for two years each; her peaceful rural life centers around this new, happy family and the big, Organic garden she grows. She religiously takes her life extension vitamins and keeps her dietary and life-style indiscretions small and infrequent. She is probably going to live a long, time.

I consider Kelly's cluster of organ weaknesses very typical of all cancers regardless of type or location, as well as being typical of AIDS and other critical infections by organisms that usually reside in the human body without causing trouble (called "opportunistic"). All these diseases are varieties of immune system failure. All of these conditions present a similar pattern of immune system weaknesses. They all center around what I call the "deadly triangle," comprised of a weak thymus gland, weak spleen, and a weak liver. The thymus and spleen form the core of the body's immune system. The weak liver contributes to a highly toxic system that further weakens the immune system. To top it off, people with cancer invariably have a poor ability to digest cooked protein (animal or vegetable) (usually from a weak pancreas unable to make enough digestive enzymes) and eat too much of it, giving them a very toxic colon, and an overloaded lymphatic system.

Whenever I analyze someone with this pattern, especially the entire deadly triangle, I let the person know that if I had those particular weaknesses I would consider my survival to be at immediate risk I'd consider it an emergency situation demanding vigorous attention. It does not matter if they don't yet have a tumor, or fibroid, or opportunistic infection; if they don't already have something of that nature they soon will.

Here's yet another example of why I disapprove of diagnosis. By giving the condition a name like "lymphoma" or "melanoma", "chronic fatigue syndrome" "Epstein-Barr syndrome" or "AIDS," "systemic yeast infection", "hepatitis" or what have, people think the doctor then understands their disease. But the doctor rarely understands that all these seemingly different diseases are essentially the same disease—a toxic body with a dysfunctional immune system. What is relevant is that a person with the deadly triangle must strengthen their immune system, and their pancreas, and their liver, and detoxify their body immediately. If these repairs are accomplished in time, the condition goes away, whatever its Latin name may have been.

Now, about some of the adjuncts to Kelly's healing. Let me stress here that had none of these substances or practices been used, she probably still would have recovered. Perhaps a bit more slowly. Perhaps a bit less comfortably. Conversely, had Kelly treated her cancer with every herb, poultice and vitamin known to man but had neglected fasting and colonics, she might well have died. It has been wisely said that intelligence may be defined as the ability to correctly determine differences, similarities, and importances. I want my readers to be intelligent about understanding the relative importances of different hygienic treatment and useful supporting practices.

Echinacea and chaparral leaves, red clover flowers, and fenugreek seeds are made into medicinal teas that I find very helpful in detoxification programs, because they all are aggressive blood or lymph cleansers and boost the immune response. These same teas can be used to help the body throw off a cold, flu, or other acute illness but they have a much more powerful effect on a fasting body than on one that is eating. Echinacea and chaparral are extraordinarily bitter and may be better accepted if ground up and encapsulated, or mixed with other teas with pleasant flavors such as peppermint or lemon grass. These teas should be simmered until they are at the strongest concentration palatable, drinking three or four cups of this concentrate a day. If you use echinacea, then chaparral probably isn't necessary and visa versa. Red clover is another blood cleanser, perhaps a little less effective but it has a pleasant, sweet taste and may be better accepted by the squeamish.

If there is lymphatic congestion I always include fenugreek seed tea brewed at the strength of approximately one tablespoon of seeds to a quart of water. Expect the tea to be brown, thick and mucilaginous, with a reasonably pleasant taste reminiscent of maple syrup.

Kelly used poultices of clay and wheat grass pulp on her lumps, somewhat like the warm castor oil poultices I used on my mother's arthritic deposits. Poultices not only feel very comforting, but they have the effect of softening up deposits and tumors so that a detoxifying, fasting body is more able to re absorb them. Poultices draw, pulling toxins out through the skin, unburdening the liver. Clay (freshly-mixed potters clay I purchase from a potters' guild), mixed with finely chopped or blended young wheat grass (in emergencies I've even used lawn grasses) makes excellent drawing poultices. Without clay, I've also used vegetable poultices made of chopped or blended comfrey leaves, comfrey root, slightly cooked (barely wilted) cabbage leaves, slightly steamed onion or garlic (cooked just enough to soften it). These are very effective to soften tumors, abscesses and ulcers. Aloe poultices are good on burns. Poultices should be thought of as helpful adjuncts to other, more powerful healing techniques and not as remedies all by themselves, except for minor skin problems.

Poultices, to be effective, need to be troweled on half an inch thick, extending far beyond the effected area, covered with cheese cloth or rags torn from old cotton sheets so they don't dry out too fast. Fresh poultices needs to be applied several times daily. They also need to be left on the body until they do dry. Then poultices are thrown away, to be followed by another as often as patience will allow. Do not cover poultices tightly with plastic because if they don't dry out they won't draw much. The drawing is in the drying.

Sometimes poultices cause a tumor or deposit to be expelled through the skin rather than being adsorbed, all with rather spectacular pus and gore. This phenomena is actually beneficial and should be welcomed because anytime the body can push toxins out through the skin, the burden on the organs of elimination are lessened.

Wheat grass juice has a powerful anti-tumor effect, is very perishable, is laborious to make, but is worth the effort because it contains powerful enzymes and nutrients that help detoxify and heal when taken internally or applied to the skin. As a last resort with dying patients who can no longer digest anything taken by mouth I've implanted wheat grass juice rectally (in a cleansed colon). Some of them haven't died. You probably can't buy wheat grass juice that retains much medicinal effect because it needs to be very fresh and should be drunk within minutes of squeezing. Chilled sharply and immediately after squeezing it might maintain some potency for an hour or two. Extracting juice from grass takes a special press that resembles a meat grinder.

The wheat is grown in transplant or seedling trays in bright light. I know someone who uses old plastic cafeteria trays for this. The seed is soaked overnight, spread densely atop a tray, covered shallowly with fine soil, kept moist but not soggy. When the grass is about four inches high, begin harvesting by cutting off the leaves with a scissors and juicing them. If the tray contains several inches of soil you usually get a second cutting of leaves. You need to start a new tray every few days; one tray can be cut for three or four days. (Kulvinskas, 1975)

More wheat grass juice is not better than just enough; three ounces a day is plenty! It is a very powerful substance! The flavor of wheat grass juice is so intense that some people have to mix it with carrot juice to get it down. DO NOT OVERUSE. The energizing effects of wheat grass can be so powerful that some people make a regular practice of drinking it. However, I've seen many people who use wheat grass juice as a tonic become allergic to it much as antibiotic dependent people do to antibiotics. Better to save wheat grass for emergencies.

I also have treated my own breast cancers–twice. The first time I was only 23 years old. One night I noticed that it hurt to sleep the way I usually did on my left side because there was a hard lump in my left breast. It was quite large–about the size of a goose egg. Having just completed RN training two years prior, I had been well brain washed about my poor prognosis and knew exactly what requisite actions must taken.

I scheduled a biopsy under anesthetic, so that if the tumor was malignant they could proceed to full mastectomy without delay. I was ignorant of any alternative course of action at the time.

I might add that before I grew my first tumor I had been consuming large amounts of red meat in a mistaken understanding gained in nursing school that a good diet contained large amounts of animal protein. In addition to the stress of being a full time psychology graduate student existing on a very low budget, I was experiencing I very frustrating relationship with a young man that left me constantly off center and confused.

A biopsy was promptly performed. The university hospital's SOP required that three pathologists make an independent decision about the nature of a tumor before proceeding with radical surgery. Two of the pathologist agreed that my tumor was malignant, which represented the required majority vote. But the surgeon removed only the lump, which he said was well encapsulated and for some reason did not proceed with a radical mastectomy. These days many surgeons routinely limit themselves to lumpectomies.

I never did find out why I awakened from general anesthetic with two breasts, but I have since supposed that due to my tender age the surgeon was reluctant to disfigure me without at least asking me for permission, or giving me some time to prepare psychologically. When I came out of anesthesia he told me that the lump was malignant, and that he had removed it, and that he needed to do a radical mastectomy to improve my prognosis over the next few years. He asked me to think it over, but he signed me up on his surgery list for the following Monday.

I did think it over and found I was profoundly annoyed at the idea of being treated like I was just a statistic, so I decided that I would be unique. I made a firm decision that I would be well and stay well–and I was for the next fifteen years. The decision healed me.

When I was 37 I had a recurrence. At the time I had in residence Ethyl and Marge, the two far-gone breast cancer cases I already told you about. I also had in residence a young woman with a breast tumor who had not undergone any medical treatment, not even a lumpectomy. (I will relate her case in detail shortly.) I was too identified emotionally with helping these three, overly-empathetic due to my own history. I found myself taking on their symptoms and their pain. I went so far into sympathy as to grow back my tumor—just as it had the first time—a lump mushroomed from nothing to the size of a goose egg in only three weeks in exactly the same place as the first one. Just out of curiosity I went in for a needle biopsy. Once again it was judged to be malignant, and I got the same pressure from the surgeon for immediate surgery. This time, however, I had an alternative system of healing that I believed in. So I went home, continued to care for my very sick residents, and began to work on myself.

The first thing I had to confront about myself was that I was being a compassionate fool. I needed to learn how to maintain my own personal boundaries, and clearly delineate what stuff in my mind and my body was really mine and what was another's. I needed to apply certain mental techniques of self-protection known to and practiced by many healers. I knew beyond doubt that I had developed sympathetic breast cancer because a similar phenomena had happened to me before. Once, when I had previously been working on a person with very severe back pain with hands-on techniques, I suddenly had the pain, and the client was totally free of it. So I protected myself when working with sick people. I would wash my hands and arms thoroughly with cold water, or with water and vinegar after contact. I would shake off their "energy," have a cold shower, walk bare foot on the grass, and visualize myself well with intact boundaries. These prophylaxes had been working for me, but I was particularly vulnerable to people with breast cancer.

I also began detoxification dieting, took more supplements, and used acupressure and reflexology as my main lines of attack. My healing diet consisted of raw food exclusively. I allowed myself fruits (not sweet fruits) and vegetables (including a lot of raw cabbage because vegetables in the cabbage family such as cauliflower and broccoli are known to have a healing effect on cancer), raw almonds, raw apricot kernels, and some sprouted grains and legumes. I drank diluted carrot juice, and a chlorophyll drink made up of wheat grass and barley green and aloe vera juice. I took echinaechia, red clover, and fenugreek seeds. I worked all the acupuncture points on my body that strengthen the immune system, including the thymus gland, lymph nodes, and spleen. I also worked the meridians, and reflex points for the liver, and large intestine. I massaged the breast along the natural lines of lymphatic drainage from the area.

Last, and of great importance, I knew that the treatment would work, and that the tumor would quickly disappear. It did vanish totally in three months. It would have gone away quicker if I had water fasted, but I was unable to do this because I needed physical strength to care for my resident patients and family.

Eighteen years have passed since that episode, and I have had no further reappearance of breast tumors. At age 55 I still have all my body parts, and have had no surgery except the original lumpectomy. Many, viewing my muscles and athletic performance, would say my health is exceptional but I know my own frailties and make sure I do not aggravate them. I still have exactly the same organ deficiencies as other cancer patients and must keep a very short leash on my lifestyle.

If for some reason I wanted to make my life very short, all I would have to do would be to abandon my diet, stop taking supplements, eat red meat and ice cream every day and be unhappy about something. Incidentally, I have had many residential clients with breast cancer since then, and have not taken on their symptoms, so I can assume that I have safely passed that hurdle.

I've helped dozens of cases of simple breast cancer where my treatment began before the cancer broadly spread. Kelly's case was not the easiest of this group, nor the hardest. Sometimes there was lymphatic involvement that the medical doctors had not yet treated in any way. All but one of my early-onset breast cancer cases recovered. I believe those are far better results than achieved by AMA treatment.

Before I crow too much, let me stress that every one of these women was a good candidate for recovery–under 40 years old, ambulatory and did not feel very sick. And most importantly, every one of them had received no other debilitating medical treatment except a needle biopsy or simple lumpectomy. None of these women had old tumors (known about for more than six months) and none of the tumors were enormous (nothing larger than a walnut).

Clearly, this group is not representative of the average breast cancer case. Hygienic therapy for cancer is a radical idea these days and tends to attract younger people, or older, desperate people who have already been through the works. In every one of my simple cases the tumors were reabsorbed by the body during the thirty days of water fasting and the client left happy.

Except one. I think I should describe this unsuccessful case, this "dirty case," so my readers get a more balanced idea of how fearsome cancer really isn't if the sick person can clearly resolve to get better and has no problem about achieving wellness.

Marie was an artisan and musician from Seattle who grew up back East in an upper-middle class dysfunctional family. She was in her late twenties. She had been sexually abused by an older brother, was highly reactive, and had never been able to communicate honestly with anyone except her lesbian lover (maybe, about some things).

Three years prior to coming to see me Marie had been medically diagnosed as having breast cancer and had been advised to have immediate surgery. She ignored this advice; Marie never told her friends, said nothing to her family and tried to conceal it from her lover because she did not want to disrupt their life together.

On her own, she did begin eating a Macrobiotic diet. In spite of this diet, the tumor grew, but grew very slowly. After two years the tumor was discovered by her lover, who after a year of exhausting and upsetting arguments, forced Marie to seek treatment. Since Marie adamantly refused to go the conventional medical route, she ended up on my doorstep as a compromise.

By this time the tumor was the size of a fist and had broken through the skin of the left breast. It was very ugly, very hard. Biokinesiology showed the usual deadly triangle and other associated organ weaknesses typical of cancer. Marie began fasting on water with colonics and poultices and bodywork and counseling and supplements. At the end of the water fast, Marie looked much healthier, with clear eyes and clear skin and had a sort of shine about her, but the tumor had only receded enough for the skin to close over it; it was still large, and very hard. To fully heal, Marie probably needed at least two more water fasts of equal length interspersed with a few months on a raw food diet. But she lacked the personal toughness to confront another fast in the near future. Nor was she emotionally up to what she regarded as the deprivation of a long-term raw foods healing diet.

So I advised her to seek other treatment. Still unwilling to accept standard medical management of her case, Marie chose to go to the Philippines to have "psychic surgery." She was excited and optimistic about this; I was interested myself because I was dubious about this magical procedure; if Marie went I would have a chance to see the results (if any) on a person I was very familiar with. Marie had her tickets and was due to leave in days when her lover, against Marie's directly-stated wishes, called her parents and informed them of what was happening.

The parents had known nothing of Marie's cancer and were shocked, upset, outraged! They had not known Marie was a lesbian, much less that their daughter was flirting with (from their view) obvious quackery. Their daughter needed immediate saving and her parents and brother (the one who had abused her) flew to Oregon and surprisingly appeared the next day in a state of violent rage. They threatened lawsuits, police, incarceration, they threatened to have their daughter civilly committed as unable to take care of herself. They thought everything Marie had done for the last three years was my fault. I was lucky to stay out of jail. Of course, all of this was why Marie had not told them in the first place; she had wanted to avoid this kind of a scene.

Marie did not have enough personal integrity to withstand the domination of her immediate family. They put her in a hospital, where Marie had a radical mastectomy, chemotherapy and radiation. Assured that they had done everything that should have been done, the self-righteous parents went back home. Marie never recovered from chemotherapy and radiation. She died in the hospital surrounded by her lesbian friends who took dedicated, ever-so-sympathetic turns maintaining an emotional round-the-clock vigil.

Marie's death was partly my fault. She was an early case of mine. At the time I did not yet understand the total effect of lack of ethics and irresponsibility on illness. Had Marie really wanted to live in the first place, she would have sought treatment three years earlier. In our counseling sessions she always evaded this question and I had not been wise enough to pin her down with my knee on her chest and make her answer up. Marie had too many secrets from everybody and was never fully honest in any of her relationships, including with me. I think she only came to Great Oaks at her lover's insistence and to the day she died was trying to pretend that nothing was wrong.

All Marie really wanted from her life was to be loved and have a lot of loving attention. In the end, her dramatic death scene gave her that, which is probably why she manifested cancer and kept it and eventually, died from it.

The name for this game is "secondary gain." A lot of sick people are playing it. Their illness lets them win their deepest desire; they get love, attention, revenge, sympathy, complete service, pampering, create guilt in others. When sick people receive too much secondary gain they never get well.

One of the hardest things about being a healer is that one accumulates an ever-enlarging series of dirty, failed cases like this one. It is depressing and makes a person want to quit doctoring. Whenever I get involved with a case I really want them to get better. My life is put entirely out of joint for several months dealing with a residential faster. My schedule is disrupted; my family life suffers; my personal health suffers. No amount of mere money could pay for this. And then some of these people go and waste all my help to accomplish some discreditable secret agenda that they have never really admitted to themselves or others.

Constant Complaints

Alice was a middle-aged woman who couldn't understand why she had always felt tired, even when she was young. Her life had been this way ever since she could remember. Most puzzling to her was why her life was so Job-like. She did everything the proper way. Doing things correctly was important to her, and fitted her Puritan background. Alice supported all the right causes, did good works, was active in a Unitarian church and bought all her food at the health food store—and made sure it was organically grown.

But in spite of Alice's righteous living, her existence was a treadmill of constant, minor complaints. She was constantly exhausted, so much so she had difficulty getting up in the morning and feared she might have chronic fatigue syndrome (whatever this is). Alice suffered bouts of depression over thoughts like these, and had many acute illnesses like colds that hung on interminably and would not go away. She had a constant post-nasal drip. Though she enjoyed life, her body was a millstone around her neck.

I've had a lot of clients exactly like Alice. Sometimes they complain of headaches; sometimes constant yeast or bladder infections. Whatever the complaints, the symptoms are rarely severe enough to classify themselves as someone who is seriously ill, but their symptoms rarely go away and they almost never feel good. Medical doctors rarely find anything wrong with them, though they will frequently prescribe an antibiotic to treat a somewhat constant infection, or an antihistamine for sinus symptoms. Getting a new prescription drug makes the complaint go away for a short time until their resistance is lowered again and the very same complaint returns. These people frequently depend on over the counter pills and are routinely prescribed sleeping remedies and antidepressants. If instead of this route they will but take my medicine they are usually easy to fix and afterwards are amazed that it was all that simple and that so much of their life has been less than it could have been.

Alice had been through the medical doctor route. She had become quite familiar with antibiotics for her colds and flu, and also took synthetic thyroid hormone–the doctor had diagnosed her fatigue as being caused by an underactive thyroid, which was partly correct–but the thyroid medication didn't give her much more energy. Alice had been supporting this medical doctor in grand style for over thirty years but never obtained the relief she sought.

I put Alice through my usual two hour first-time-visit thorough analysis. For two weeks before coming to see me she had saved tiny samples of everything she ate, wrapped them in plastic film, carefully labeled, and put them in the freezer. Along with these food samples and a typed list of all these foods, she brought a big box full of her condiments, herb teas, vitamins, spices, prescription medications, over the counter drugs, oils, grains, breads, crackers and small samples of her usual fresh vegetables and fruits. Even her water. Her entire kitchen! By biokinesiology we proceeded to test all of her foods for allergic reactions. I also tested the integrity of her organs and glands and in the process, got a detailed medical history and list of her complaints.

Alice had exhausted adrenals, and they probably had been that way for thirty years. Her pancreas was now too weak to digest the legumes that made up a large part of her vegetarian diet. She was allergic to wheat, soy, and dairy products and had especially been eating dairy in the mistaken notion that it was necessary to keep up her protein intake. Really very typical. So many health food store shoppers these days mistakenly believe that, because they are vegetarian and do not eat meat, they especially need to boost their protein intake with dairy and soy. Unfortunately, so many North Americans are highly allergic to dairy and unfortunately, soy products are as hard or harder to digest than cooked meats.

Alice was especially shocked to discover that she was allergic to such foods as cabbage family vegetables, alfalfa sprouts and citrus. Most people don't think that anyone could be allergic to something as healthy as alfalfa sprouts. The doctor was right about one thing; her thyroid was underperforming. He had not noticed that her heart was weak.

Medical doctors rarely discover an organ weakness until that organ actually begins to catastrophically fail. A busy honest doctor will usually tell the complaining patient there is nothing wrong with them: go home, take two aspirin, accept the fact that your body is not perfect and don't worry about it. A hungry doctor will be delighted to perform countless lab tests, seeking any possible reason for the complaint. This can go on as long as the patient has money or as long as the insurance company will pay. They rarely find anything "wrong" and the patient is far better off if the doctor doesn't discover something "serious" to treat because their treatment may carry with it consequences far more severe than the complaint. For example, I have seen dozens of people whose lives were virtually ruined after surgical treatment for chronic back pain.

Biokinesiology is actually a far more sensitive system of analysis than lab tests. It picks up weaknesses at a very early stage so total organ failure can be prevented. Rarely will any of the organ weaknesses I discover be confirmed by a medical doctor. First I put Alice on a six week cleanse. She did one week on fresh, raw food; one week on dilute carrot juice with some green leafy vegetables juice too; one week on water fasting; and then she repeated the series. After six weeks of detoxification, I gave Alice a life extension megavitamin formula, discovered she could not handle the acid form of vitamin C (that she had already been taking) and had her start on protomorphogens to rebuild her weakened endocrine system, her exhausted adrenals and weak pancreas. She also began taking pancreatic enzymes when she ate vegetable protein. She was put on a maintenance diet that eliminated foods she was allergic to; the diet primarily consisted of whole grains, nuts, cooked and raw vegetables, and raw fruits. On her maintenance diet Alice had a profound resurgence of energy and rediscovered a sense of well-being she had not known for decades. She began to feel like she had when she was a child. Her constant sinus drip was gone. She was able to stop taking synthetic thyroid hormones and instead, supported her endocrine system with protomorphogens.

A Rampaging Infection

At the age of 40, John, an old bohemian client of mine, came into a moderate inheritance and went "native" in the Fiji Islands in the South Pacific. He spent about four months hanging out with the locals. Life there was so much fun that John completely forgot that his body was actually rather delicate, that many of his organs were weak, and that to feel good, he had to live a fairly simon-pure life.

But the jovial, accepting, devil-may-care Fijians enjoyed a constant party, even more so because John's money allowed the Fijians to manifest powerful, tropical, home-grown strains of recreational herbs to smoke in abundance, beer and rum and worse, the Fijians (and John) constantly used a very toxic though only mildly-euphoric narcotic called kava, something Europeans usually have no genetic resistance to. The Fijians (and John) also ate a lot of freshly-caught fish fried in grease, well-salted, and huge, brain-numbing bowls of greasy starches, foods that they call i'coi, or "real food" as opposed to things like fruit and vegetables that aren't real food because they don't knock you to the floor for hours trying to digest them in a somnambulant doze.

John miraculously kept up with this party for a few months and then, while scuba diving, got some small coral scratches on his leg. These got infected. The infections got worse. Soon he had several huge, suppurating, ulcerous sores on his legs and worse, the infections became systemic and began spreading rapidly. He was running a fever and was in considerable pain. So John booked an emergency ticket home and fled to find Doctor Isabelle. When I met his plane he was rolled out in a wheelchair, unable to walk because of pain and swelling in his legs.

John was violently opposed to ordinary medical treatment; he especially would not have taken antibiotics even if he had died without them because previous courses of antibiotics had been the precipitant of life-threatening conditions that first brought John to my care. John used his last strength to get to me because he knew that had a hospital gotten its clutches on him the medical doctors would have done exactly as they pleased.

I gave John a colonic, a gentle, mental spanking, and put him to bed without any supper. He started water fasting and did colonics every day. He began gobbling vitamin C (as calcium ascorbate) a few grams every hour. I put huge poultices on his sores made of clay and chopped lawn grass (we needed a week or so before a tray of wheat grass would be ready). John's sores were amazing. Every day a new one seemed to appear on a different part of the body. The old ones kept getting bigger and deeper. The largest original ones were about three inches in diameter, smelled horribly and had almost eaten the flesh down to the bone. His pain was severe; there was no position John could assume that didn't irritate one sore or another, and it was a good thing my house was remote because John frequently relieved his pain by screaming. John was never delirious, but he was always original. He did not have to scream, but enjoyed its relief and howled quite dramatically. I wore earplugs.

After about two weeks of water fasting, John counted up the total of his sores. There were forty three. Seven or eight of them were enormous, two or three inches in diameter and well into the flesh, but the last ones to appear were shallow, small and stayed small. After that point no more new ones showed up and the body began to make visible headway against the infection. Very slowly and then more and more rapidly, the sores began to close up and heal from the edges. John's fever began to drop.

And he had less pain. I should mention that John brought an extremely virulent and aggressive pathogenic organism into our house to which we Americans had no resistance. Both my husband and I were attacked where the skin had been broken. However, unlike John, in our cases, our healthy bodies immediately walled-off the organism and the small, reddened pustules, though painful, did not grow and within a week, had been conquered by our immune systems. And after that we had an immunity.

After about three weeks of his fasting we were thoroughly tired of hearing John's cathartic howls, tired of nursing a sick person. We needed a break. John at this point could walk a bit and was feeling a lot better. John had previously water fasted for 30 days and knew the drill very well. So we stocked up the vitamin C bottle by his bed and went to town for the weekend to stay in a motel and see a movie. As they say in the Canadian backwoods, we were bushed.

John had promised to be good. But as soon as we left he decided that since he felt so very much better, he could break his fast. He knew how to do this and fortunately for him, (it was very much premature for John to eat) did it more or less correctly, only eating small quantities of raw fruits and vegetables. But by the time we got back home three days later, John had relapsed. The pain was rapidly getting much worse; the sores were growing again and a few small new ones appeared. Dr. Isabelle again took away his food and gave him another verbal spanking a little more severe than the one he'd had a few weeks earlier and put him to bed again without his supper.

After two more weeks on water, John had gained a great deal on the sores. They were filling in and weren't oozing pus, looked clean and the new forming meat looked a healthy pink instead of purple-black. But John had been very slender to start with and by now he was getting near the end of his food reserves. He probably couldn't have fasted on water for more than one more week without starvation beginning. But this time, when he broke his fast, it was under close supervision. I gave him dilute juice only, introduced other sustenance very cautiously and made absolutely sure that reintroducing nourishment would not permit the organism to gain. This time it didn't. John's own immune system, beefed up by fasting, had conquered a virulent organism that could have easily killed him.

Before the era of antibiotics, before immunizations to the common childhood illnesses, people frequently died of infections as virulent as the one that attacked John. They usually died because they "ate to keep up their strength." Most of these deaths were unnecessary, caused by ignorance and poor nursing care. For example, standard medical treatment for typhoid fever used to consist of spoon-fed milk—sure to kill all but the strongest constitution. Even without the assistance of massive doses of vitamin C, if people would but fast away infections they could cure themselves of almost all of them with little danger, without the side effects of antibiotics or creating mutated antibiotic-resistant strains of bacteria.

Dr. John Tilden, a hygienist who practiced in the '20s, before the era of antibiotics, routinely fasted patients with infectious illnesses. Supporting the sick body with wise nursing, he routinely healed scarlet fever, whopping cough, typhoid, typhus, pneumonia, peritonitis, Rocky Mountain fever, tuberculosis, gonorrhea, syphilis, cholera, and rheumatic fever. The one common infection he could not cure was diphtheria involving the throat. (Tilden, Impaired Health, Vol. II).

Recently, medical gerontologists have discovered another reason that fasting heals infections. One body function that deteriorates during the aging process is the production of growth hormone so the effects of growth hormone have been studied. This hormone also stimulates the body to heal wounds and burns, repair broken bones, generally replace any tissues that have been destroyed and, growth hormone stimulates the immune response. Growth hormone also maintains muscle tone and its presence generally slows the aging process.

Growth hormone might make a wonderful life-extension supplement; on it a middle-aged person might readily maintain the muscle tone of youth while slowing aging in general. Unfortunately, growth hormone cannot at this time be inexpensively synthesized and is still far too costly to be used therapeutically except to prevent dwarfism. However, any technique that encourages a body to produce more of this hormone would be of great interest to life extensionists.

The body only produces growth hormone at certain times and only when certain nutrients are present in the blood. Gerontologists call these nutrients "precursors." The precursors are two essential amino acids, argenine and ornithine and certain vitamins such as C and B6. But having the precursors present is not enough. Growth hormone is only manufactured under certain, specific circumstances: for about one hour immediately after going to sleep and then only if the blood supply is rich with argenine and ornithine but contains few other amino acids; it is also manufactured during heavy aerobic exercise that goes on for more than thirty minutes; and growth hormone is produced at an accelerated rate when fasting. (Pearson and Shaw, 1983). I did not know this when I was fasting John, but now, I would give argenine and ornithine to someone with a serious infection as well as massive quantities of vitamin C.

Chronic Back Pain

Barry was a carpenter who couldn't afford to lose work because he was unable to bend or twist or lift. He frequently had bouts of severe back pain that made working almost impossible. Upon analysis by biokinesiology I found that he had a major problem with large intestine weakness and secondarily, adrenal weakness.

Constipation frequently causes back pain. The muscles of the back have nerve pathway connections to the large intestines; weakness in the intestine causes weakness of the back and makes it prone to injury. But the problem is the intestine, not the back. And the only way to make the back stay better is to heal the intestine. Many athletes have very similar problems. For example, they get knee injuries and think there is something wrong with their knee. Or they get shoulder injuries and think their shoulder is weak. These people are only half right. Yes, their knee or their shoulder is weak. But it could become strong and almost uninjurable if the underlying cause of the weakness is corrected.

The knee for example, has nerve pathway connections to the adrenal glands and kidneys. The shoulder has similar connections to the thyroid. The foot is weakened by the bladder. The treatment should first be on the weakened gland or organ and secondarily, on the damaged muscle tissue. I have solved numerous sports-related knee problems with protomorphogens for the adrenals and elimination of food allergies that make the adrenals work overtime. I have fixed bad shoulders by rebuilding the thyroid.

In Barry's case, it was the intestine. I asked him about his bowel function and he said that he was never constipated, had "a daily bowel movement without a lot of straining." But having given some 6,000 colonics, I knew better. There should have been no straining; Barry was trying very hard to be regular–he should not have had to effort. Fortunately, it struck him as true that he needed to detoxify and I managed to convince him to water fast. He probably figured, why not since he couldn't work anyway. Barry was a tall, skinny man to start with and you would think he hardly carried any fat at all, but he fasted on water for 30 days, receiving a colonic every day, while I did bodywork on his damaged back. He sure was constipated and couldn't deny the evidence that floated by through the sight tube of the colonic machine. By the end of the fast his colon was fairly repaired and free of old fecal material. And Barry had become a tall, gaunt-looking guy who had lost about 20 pounds you wouldn't think he had to spare.

After a few weeks of careful weaning back on to food, Barry felt pretty good, terrific even. He had no back pain and found out for the first time what not being constipated meant. It no longer took "not very much effort" to move his bowels; they moved themselves. That was ten years ago. A few months ago, Barry looked me up, just to say thanks and to let me know that he had not had any more back problems and had generally felt good because he had more or less stayed on the improved diet I had instructed him about during his fast.

Painful Menstruation

Elsie was twenty. She came to see me because I had helped Elsie's mother overcome breast cancer many years earlier. Elsie began to have very painful periods with profuse bleeding and abdominal pain. Her nutrition had been generally good because her mother couldn't survive on the average American diet and had long ago converted her family to vegetarianism. And like her mother, Elsie had been taking vitamins for many years.

A medical doctor diagnosed Elsie as having endometriosis, meaning, the lining of her uterus had migrated to the fallopian tubes, where it continued to bleed regularly into the abdominal cavity, following the same hormonal cycle as the endometrital tissue that lines the uterus. The doctor offered to try hormonal manipulation and if this proved unsuccessful, offered a hysterectomy. That would certainly eliminate the symptoms!

But Elsie did not wish to eliminate her ability to have children and preferred not to risk throwing her hormones off balance. So she came to me. My analysis showed that she had weak ovaries and weak uterus. These were secondary to a toxic colon, toxic because she had a weak gall bladder and weak pancreas that reduced her digestive capacity and turned her improperly combined Organic, vegetarian legume-rich diet into toxemia. Checking her foods for allergies I discovered the normal pattern: Elsie was intolerant to dairy, wheat, eggs, corn, soy and concentrated sugars.

Being no stranger to fasting (her mother had fasted at length ten years previously) Elsie undertook a 30 day cleanse on vegetable juice with daily enemas, taking vitamins in powdered form. After the fast I put her on protomorphogens for her reproductive organs and pancreas. The gall bladder had healed by itself during fasting–gall bladders usually heal easily. Her maintenance diet included using pancreatic enzyme supplements when eating vegetable proteins and Elsie eliminated most fats so her gall bladder would not be stressed. The fasting also overcame her allergic reactions to corn and wheat but she was still unable to handle soy products, eggs or dairy. After six months Elsie no longer needed protomorphogens, had no abdominal pain and her periods were normal.

You may well be wondering how or why detoxification of the bowels allowed the body to repair the uterus. The large intestine is a sort of nest that cradles the reproductive organs, including the ovaries, uterus, and in the case of the male, the prostate gland. A toxic colon is like having one rotten apple in a basket, it contaminates the whole batch. Many problems in the abdominal area are caused by a toxic colon, including chronic back pain, ovarian cysts, infertility, birth abnormalities, bladder infections and bladder cancer, painful menstruation, fibroids and other benign growths as well as malignant ones, and prostatitis or prostate cancer. Detoxing the body and cleaning out the colon should be a part of the healing of all of these conditions.

Irritable Bowels

Some peoples' lives don't run smoothly. Jeanne's certainly didn't. She was abandoned to raise three little kids on welfare. Her college diploma turned out to be useless. Jeanne used to help me at Great Oaks in exchange for treatment. During those early years she had done a 30 day juice fast with colonics. Twenty years later at age 60, having survived three children's growing up, surviving the profound, enduring loss of one who died as an adult, after starting up and running a small business that for many years barely paid its way, and experiencing an uninsured fire that took her house, she began to develop abdominal pains the doctors named "irritable bowel syndrome" or "colitis." The MD offered antibiotics and antispasmodics but Jeanne had no insurance, the remedies were unaffordable. She also retained considerable affinity for natural medicine.

Prior to these symptoms her diet had been vegetarian, and had included large quantities of raw fruits and vegetables and whole grains. But the bran in bread was irritating to her bowels, she could no longer digest raw vegetables or most raw fruit.

Jeanne's vital force was low; her healing took time. She started on a long fast supported by powdered vitamins, vegetable broth and herb teas, but after three weeks was too weak to do her own enemas at home and could not shop for vegetables to cook into broth. So she had to add one small serving of cooked vegetable per day, usually broccoli or steamed kale. This lasted for one more week but Jeanne, having no financial reserves, had to return to work, and needed to regain energy quickly. Though not totally healed, she progressed to a maintenance diet of cooked grains and vegetables and food supplements, very much like a Macrobiotic diet. She felt better for awhile but wore down again after another stressful year.

Her abdominal pains gradually returned though this time she noticed they were closely associated with her stresses. About one year after ending her first fast, as soon as she could arrange to take time off, she began another. This time to avoid extreme weakness, she took vegetable broth from the outset, as well as small amounts of carrot juice and one small serving of cooked vegetable a day for three weeks. Again, this rest allowed the digestive tract to heal and the pain went away. She returned to her Macrobiotic diet with selected raw foods that she could now handle without irritating her bowel.

She was now healthier then she had been in many years. With improved energy and a more positive attitude, Jeanne returned to University at age 65 and obtained a teaching certificate. Now she is making good money, doing work she enjoys for the first time in 35 years. I hope she has a long and happy life. She is entitled to one!

A Collection of Gallbladders

Gallbladder cases are rather ho-hum to me; they are quick to respond to hygienic treatment and easy to resolve. I've fixed lots of them. But an inflamed gallbladder is in no way ho-hum to the person afflicted with it. I've been frequently told that there are no worse pains a body can create than an inflamed gallbladder or the sensations accompanying the passing of a gall stone. I hear from kidney patients that passing a kidney stone is worse but I've never had a patient who experienced both kinds of stones to give me an honest comparative evaluation.

The only thing dangerous about simple gallbladder problems is ignoring them (between the bouts of severe pain they can cause) because then the inflamed gallbladder can involve the liver. I already told the story of how my own mother lost half her liver this way.

The condition is usually caused by a combination of hereditary tendency, general toxemia, and/or a high-fat diet, especially one high in animal fats. The liver makes bile that is stored in the gallbladder, to be released on demand into the small intestine to digest fat. A toxic, overloaded liver makes irritating sediment-containing bile that inflames the gallbladder and forms stones. A high-fat diet forces the liver to make even more of this irritant.

A toxic, overloaded, inflamed, blocked gallbladder is capable of causing an enormous array of symptoms that can seem to have no connection at all to their cause. In part these same symptoms are caused by a toxic, constipated colon that, in part, got that way because of poor fat digestion over a long time. These symptoms include: severe back pain; headache; bloating; burping; nausea; insomnia; intestinal gas; generalized aches and pains.

Medical doctors used to remove a troublesome gallbladder without hesitation; it was an organ they considered to be highly dispensable. Without one, the bile duct takes over as a bladder but its capacity is much smaller so the person's ability to digest fats has been permanently crippled, leading to increased toxemia and earlier aging if fats are not eliminated from the diet. These days the medicos have a new, less invasive procedure to eliminate stones; they are vibrated and broken-up by ultrasonics without major surgery. Inflamed gallbladders are usually removed because gallbladder inflammations resist treatment by antibiotics.

There are several very effective natural gallbladder remedies. The best is a three week fast, taking the juice of one or two lemons every day, along with colonics. The lemon juice tends to clear the bile duct. The fast allows the gallbladder to heal from inflammation. In cases that aren't too severe I have had very good results simply eliminating fats from the diet and using a food supplement derived from beet tops called AF Betafood. However, in all these cases, once the gallbladder is no longer "acting up," the person must stay on a low fat diet. Any fats they do eat must be vegetable and in small quantities.

By healing their gallbladders and cleansing their colons, several of my clients have resolved severe, debilitating back pain, pain so severe that the suffers were becoming bedridden. Medical doctors don't associate gallbladder disease with back pain.

The Frightening Heart

Heart disease is one of the major causes of death among North Americans. It evokes images of resuscitation, of desperate races against time, trying to restart an arrested heart before the brain dies. It makes people think of horribly expensive surgery, last wills and testaments, terrible, paralyzing pain. Heart disease is a great profit center for the medical profession.

Most heart problems are very easy to fix by holistic approaches, even many hereditary weaknesses and malfunctions can be healed, if the work is done before too much organic damage occurs. But it rarely is easy to get the people to take the necessary medicine; everything in their lives must change—and fast.

First of all, people with heart problems must rapidly reach and maintain normal weight. This can be done by fasting or by dietary change, usually by eliminating all fats, sugars and refined starches. Alcohol and tobacco must instantly and forever become only past memories. It is almost as essential to eliminate flesh protein foods and dairy. Should that prove entirely too painful, fish in small quantities and only one or two times a week is tolerable.

For starters, a long fast, especially one involving lots of bed rest, is ideal. This gives the heart a chance to heal while the body weight is adjusted. A period of intense rest even without water fasting will accomplish almost as much. Even someone with the potential for heart disease who has not yet had a heart attack would be well-served to spend a month in bed, losing weight on juice, or sitting in a rocker on the porch eating only raw foods. After the weight is down to normal or close to normal and the heart tests stronger, an exercise program should be started.

Exercise has to become a religion. A daily aerobic program must be started on a carefully managed gradient, using the pulse rate as an regulator, at first raising their maximum heart rate to a point just below 150 percent of its resting pulse and keeping it there for thirty minutes. One can walk, jog, ride a bicycle or use an exercise machine. Actually, everyone should do this, even those with no heart problems. My husband, who hates the boredom of exercise, enjoys a ski machine in front of the TV while the stock market program is on. He finds the TV interesting enough that he pays no attention to his workout. Daily aerobic exercise will strengthen the heart, gradually slowing the heart's resting pulse rate, indicating that the heart has become much stronger, pumping more blood with each pulse. As the resting pulse drops the exercising heartbeat can be increased to double the resting rate.

Highly aggressive, competitive, stress-oriented people have to give up being adrenaline junkies and learn to relax and assume a laid-back approach to living. Or die soon. An adrenaline junkie is someone that enjoys the feeling they get when operating under stress. Stress and the adrenaline it releases produce a kind of a drug-high. Many stressaholics cannot give up their adrenaline addiction while maintaining their previous employment and life-style, even though their life is at stake. In this sense they are like alcoholics, who should not take employment tending bar. To survive for long these people may have to retire or change professions. Stockbrokers may have to become Organic farmers; journalists may have to operate a news stand or bookstore, or work part-time covering the society page and dog shows. Women frequently turn their family life into a stress-filled drama too.

With heart problems a life extension megavitamin program is essential, even for twenty somethings if they have heart disease. The sixty milligrams of Co-Enzyme Q-10 I recommend for the average middle aged person will not be enough for heart cases; they should take at least 120 milligrams daily and consider up to 250 mg. This much Q-10 greatly boosts the energy output of the heart on a cellular level. Vitamin E should also be increased, to between 600 and 2,000 iu daily. I also rebuild diseased hearts with protomorphogens; usually they must stay on protomorphogens for the rest of their lives. Niacin taken several times a day in doses, sufficient to dilate the capillaries and cause a skin flush (50 to 200 milligrams), increases the blood flow to nourish the heart. The amino acid L. Carnitine is also useful by increasing the energy output of the heart much like Co-Enzyme Q-10.

When I put people on this program, the supplements and other measures gradually take effect, and over months the patient begins to feel enormously better. Inevitably they come to dislike the side-effects of the various medications their medical doctor has put them on and they begin to wean themselves off of heart-stimulating poisons like digitalis. Another benefit of my program is that inevitably, blood pressure also drops to a normal range so if they have been on blood pressure medication they quit that too. Their diuretics also become unnecessary. The money they save more than pays for their supplements and the sense of well-being they feel is beyond value.

Other Kinds *of* Cancer

There seem to be many other kinds of cancer, at least if you believe the medical doctors. They divide up cancers and their treatments by their location in the body and by the type of cancer cells present. I do not see it that way. To me, a cancer is a cancer is a cancer, and there is only one kind: it is an immune system collapse, consequence of the deadly triangle of weak spleen, thymus and liver, plus a toxic large intestine and weak pancreas. That organ profile is found in skin cancer, prostate cancer, leukemia, brain cancer, cancer of what have you. How fast or how slowly the cells multiply or spread, where they are located, what the cancer cells look like in a microscope, these are irrelevant factors compared to the body's ability to conquer the disease. Or die from it.

If the body's immune system can stop the growth of the cancers and begin to turn them back before the cancer cells impinge catastrophically on some vital function, the person can usually survive. Even if the body cannot completely eliminate all the cancer cells, but regains enough immune function to keep the existing cancers in permanent check, a person can survive many years with an existing, stable cancer without undue pain or discomfort. Still having a non-growing tumor after a long fast indicates that a person is a lot better than they were before fasting.

I believe that virtually everyone has cancer cells in their body, just like viruses and bacteria. But most people do not develop cancer as a disease because their immune function is strong so these misbehaving cells are destroyed as fast as they appear. Mutated, freely-multiplying cells are caused by peroxidized fats, by free radicals in the body, by radiation (there has always been background radiation on Earth), by chance mutation. There are naturally occurring highly carcinogenic substances in ordinary foods that are unavoidable. In fact some of these naturally occurring substances are far more dangerous than the toxic residues of pesticides in our foods. The body is supposed to deal with all these things; they are all called insults. It is rarely the insult, but the failure of the body to eliminate cancerous cells promptly that causes the disease called cancer. So the treatment I recommend for cancer in general is the same as the one described for breast cancer cases. Restore the immune function.

However, as much as I lack respect for conventional medical cancer therapies, I do think surgery can have a useful place in cancer treatment along with hygienic methods. Some people just cannot confront the lump(s). Or they are so terrified of having a cancer in their body that their emotions suppresses their own immune function. Even though surgery prompts a cancer to spread more rapidly, without their lumps some cancer patients feel more positive. If surgery is done in conjunction with rebuilding the immune system, the body will prevent new cancers from forming.

Removal of a large mass of cancer cells can also lighten the immune system's task. Not having to kill off and reabsorb all those cells one-by-one from a huge cancer mass, the body can better conquer smaller groups of cancer cells. And the die-off of large cancers produces a lot of toxins, burdening the organs of elimination. This is an argument for the potential benefit of a lumpectomy. However, I do not support mastectomies, or the type of surgery that cause massive damage to the body in a foolish attempt to remove every last cancer cell, as though the cells themselves were the disease.

Sometimes cancer tumors are well-encapsulated, walled off and can be easily removed without prompting metastasis. This type of tumor may not be completely reabsorbed by the body in any case; though the immune system may have killed it, an empty shell remains, like a peanut shell. Sometimes the judgment calls about surgery can get dicey. When surgery involves removing an organ. I oppose the loss of useful body parts.

I have also known and helped people who believed they couldn't recover without radiation and chemotherapy. What people believe is, is. The emotions generated when a personal reality is suppressed, ignored or invalidated will overwhelm an immune system. I always tell those people who sincerely believe in it to go ahead with standard medical treatment (while I'm privately praying the doctors won't cause too much damage). However, when I am supporting a body with supplements and dietary reform, have put that body on a raw-food cleansing diet or even a raw food diet with nuts and grains that hardly detoxifies, and then the person has had chemotherapy and radiation, the medical doctors in attendance are inevitably amazed that the side effects are much milder than anticipated, or non-existent. And fewer courses of chemotherapy are needed than the doctors expected.

For example, I worked with a little boy with leukemia. His mother brought him to me while trying to resolve a conflict with her ex-husband about the boy's treatment. The father demanded the standard medical route; the mother was for natural therapy. Eventually the father won in court, but I had the boy on my program for three months before the doctors got their hands on him. Even during chemotherapy and radiation the mother kept the boy on my program. Throughout the doctors' treatment he had so few bad side effects that he was able to continue in school and play with the other children; he did not lose his hair (which would have made him feel like a freak). He recovered. I don't mind that the medical doctors took credit, but to my thinking, he recovered despite their therapy.

Onion Cases

All too many of my cases are what I privately refer to as onion cases. By this I mean the opposite of a simple case. There are multiple complaints. I call them onion cases because these people get better in layers, like pealing an onion. As each skin comes off, the next becomes visible. Sometimes when the patient overcomes an existing complaint, another appears that was not there in the beginning, probably this new one is a complaint that they had at an earlier point in their life, one that had gone away. Onion cases take a long time to completely heal, sometimes years. There frequently are psychological aspects to the case that surface with different physical problems. If I were not an effective psychologist I could not succeed with most of them. The average medical doctor probably considers onion cases to be hypochondriacs, but they usually are not.

Almost always the first symptoms that demand attention are the most life-threatening, like immune system failures, liver failures, pancreatic failures, nervous system failures and heart failures. With these eliminated, new complaints appear. Often these are endocrine system imbalances or weak endocrine glands, anemias, mild heart conditions. Then it gets down to eye or ear infections, muscular or skeletal weaknesses, mild skin problems, sinusitis, teeth problems; things that aren't serious but that do degrade the quality of life. Each one of these layers also carries with it a psychological component; each of these layers can take three to six months to resolve.

I had a pretty good idea from the first visit that Daniel, not yet 30, was going to take some time to get well. He already had a degenerative condition not usually seen until middle age–crippling gout and arthritis. He had badly distorted joints, walked with considerable pain, lacked a full range of movement, had enormous fatigue and consequently, a well-justified depression. Daniel was about to give up working as no longer possible, but he liked his job. And he certainly needed it.

Daniel's analysis showed massive allergies to foods, a systemic yeast and multiple virus infections and multiple organ weaknesses: a life-threateningly weak immune system, weak pancreas, weak adrenals, weak large intestine. Because he could hardly accept anything he wasn't allergic to and because he could not afford to quit working even for a few weeks (though he was about to be forced into complete disability) I put him on a Bieler fast. This is a monodiet of fairly substantial quantities of either well-cooked green beans or well-cooked zucchini, the choice between these two foods depending on the acid-base balance of the blood. (Henry Bieler, 1965) In Daniel's case my choice was zucchini, one pint of plain zucchini puree with a little kelp and garlic added (no salt, no butter, no nothing else) every few hours. I also put him on heavy vitamin support and protomorphogens for his desperate immune system. While on the Bieler fast he did daily enemas at home. Had colonics been available to him, Daniel couldn't have afforded them.

Within three weeks he was far more comfortable, had less pain, more energy even though he was still eating nothing but zucchini, had less swelling in his joints. During the first month he lost about ten pounds and had been skinny to start with. I then added other cooked nonstarchy vegetables to his diet and we continued the same protomorphogen and supplement program for another month.

Once each month Daniel came to see me. Each time he had slightly improved organ strength and was able to tolerate a few more foods. By the third month he stopped losing weight because we added small quantities of cooked rice and millet to his diet. However, to continue his detox, I had him water fast one day a week, staying in bed and resting all day. At the start and end of the fasting day he also took an enema. He continued a weekly one-day fast for many months. By the fourth month, his immune system testing stronger, a new problem appeared. Daniel had intestinal parasites. So I also put him on a six month program to eliminate those.

Daniel required monthly dietary adjustments because he quickly became allergic if he ate very much of anything very often–broccoli or rice for example. During this time he became aware of many negative emotions associated with childhood, of young adult frustrations and disappointments. He was really very angry about many things in his life, even though he had for many years maintained an invariably pleasant social veneer. But now he began expressing some of these feelings to me and to his associates.

Daniel had an abusive girlfriend, but as he improved this relationship became insufferable. So he broke off with this woman and found a new relationship that was much more positive, one based on mutual respect and admiration. There are frequently strong connections between repressed anger and depository diseases like arthritis and gout. Daniel could not permit himself to constantly be made angry and still get well.

His next layer of symptoms did not appear until nearly eighteen months after he had first come to see me. By this time he had good energy, had returned to hiking and skiing, camping and canoeing. He had worked as a printer but was now bootstrapping his own print shop on a shoestring, and became entirely self-employed. He had a good romantic relationship. The parasites were gone; his gout and arthritis was virtually gone; many of his food allergies were gone. Now his body was demanding that its acid/base balance be adjusted and he began to pay attention to the minor back problems he had all along. Daniel had also developed a new problem–inflammation of the eye. It was so severe that he went to an opthamologist seeking immediate relief because he could hardly see. I put him on massive doses of vitamin C and protomorphogens for the eye and we attacked the other problems.

Now I still see Daniel every three months for minor dietary and supplement adjustments. His emotional space is very positive. His business is doing well. His love life is doing well. He has developed no new problems and all the old ones are under control. His organ systems, though better, will never tolerate many insults, physical or mental, but if he lives within his limits, he has every chance of a long and happy life.

Daniel has become a friend of mine by now and I like to see him but I expect I won't see Daniel very much at all any more. He has learned what he needs to know to take care of himself. This is a typical onion case that resolved successfully. However this case might not have worked out so well had Daniel not possessed a high degree of personal integrity and bravery, had he not faced and resolved his emotional conflicts. Fortunately, Daniel had always conducted an ethical life, without dishonesty or a secret collection of disreputable acts. Bodies are easy to fix; they are carbon oxygen engines that work on chemistry and respond unfailingly to physical measures. But the entity that runs the body is not so simple. The thoughts and emotions of the spirit impinge on a body as powerfully or more powerfully than all the vitamins, dietary reform or protomorphogens I can provide. The mind, and the spirit behind that mind, can make a body sick or can prevent it from getting well or staying well despite everything I do.

Unethical Illness

I see a lot of spiritually-induced physical illness in my practice. Maybe more than my share. Maybe its karmic; it tends to find me because I understand it. And it comes up my driveway because people who have it often become doctor shoppers, and seek out a naturopath as a last resort after exhausting everything that modern medical science has to offer. I have had large numbers of undiagnosable people that suffer greatly but who medical doctors can find nothing wrong with and label psychosomatic. I have also repaired people given specific medical diagnoses that standard physical remedies cannot make better.

In most of these cases, the physical illness is secondary to, is an overlay of a more fundamental spiritual cause. On this type of case there are inevitably severe problems connected with close friends, relatives and business associates. The sick person inevitably blames the friends, relatives and business associates and takes no responsibility. The problems seem unresolvable. When I probe deeply enough into these problems, I begin to discover the real infection below. The sick person, so fond of complaining about all the terrible things done to them by the people they have or have had problems with, or sometimes, so proud of not complaining about all the terrible things done to them. Actually, almost inevitably this person has committed a huge mass of secret crimes, viciousness and betrayals, rarely indictable felonious acts, but crimes none the less, disreputable deeds that must be kept secret.

These deeds are always completely justified; the sick person always claims to have been right for having done them and it is next to impossible for me as a therapist to get them to take responsibility for their sins. But at the deep, center of almost all people is an honest, decent soul that knows what it has really done and feels guilty and judges itself. That is why it says in the Bible, 'judge not, lest you be judged'. It is not the judgment of the Deity we have so much to fear; we are own worst judge, jury, and executioner, and eventually extract from ourselves full payment with compound interest for all harmful acts.

People frequently punish themselves with severe, incapacitating illness or even death. A spiritual illness will not respond very well to physical treatment until the spiritual malaise's is resolved. This case has to find enough courage to become honest with themselves, to admit their deeds in all their disgusting detail and then to make amends, or if amends are not possible, to at least cease and desist. They have to take personal responsibly for what they really are being and what they have really done and most importantly, accept that they are responsible for creating their own illness. It is not a virus, a cancer cell or something that just fell out of the universe and struck them, innocent victims that they are. They have made their illness and only they can uncreate it.

Unfortunately, few people who have spent a lifetime indulging themselves in this degree of irresponsibility have the integrity to change. This is a tough case. Especially so because they think they are physically ill, they did not come to me to be defined as a "mental" case and tend to reject such approaches.

There is no shortage of additional degenerative conditions that I could describe. There are eating disorders, shingles, skin problems, kidney disease, Alzheimer's, senility, mental illness, addictions, chronic fatigue syndrome, aids. There's macular degeneration, carpal tunnel syndrome, chronic ear infections (especially in children), tonsillitis, bronchitis, pancreatitis, cystitis, urethritis, prostatitis, colitis, sinusitis, osteomyelitis and a dozen other itises, including appendicitis. There's algias (itises of the nerves): neuralgia, fibromyalgia. There's ism's (really itises of the muscles). There are 'onias like pneumonia; omas like carcinoma, melanoma and lymphoma.

I could (but won't) write a page or two on every one of these conditions and turn this book into an encyclopedia. After twenty five years of practice, there is little I have not seen. Or helped a body repair. Generally, everyone of those following pages I'm not going to bother to write would repeat the same message. That the medical profession has little understanding of the real causes or cures of disease; that the world is full of unnecessary suffering; that there are simple, painless, effective, harmless approaches to eliminating most of the ailments of mankind except the ultimate ailment, old age, the thing that takes us all eventually; that essentially all the diseases resolve from the same approach.

But I have already explained the theoretical basis of natural hygiene, the key role of toxemia, enervation, constipation, the essentials of good diet, fasting and colon cleansing, the importance of regular exercise, and the rational for vitamin supplementation. I have revealed a lot of the secrets in my bag of tricks, like my favorite herbs, poultices and wheat grass.

What concerns me most about medicine today is that there seems to be ever fewer hygienists practicing. The young holistic practitioner is overwhelmed with confusing data and approaches and is increasingly less able to discern what is really important and what is distraction, and is increasingly intimidated by the AMA, made fearful of accepting people with serious conditions. Too many young practitioners become ideologues, clinging to the rightness of a single rigid discipline, missing the truths that exist in other approaches and worse, missing the limitations that exist in their own personal healing methods.

The current concern about the cost of medical care and resorting to government-run insurance programs and regulations will do little or nothing to reverse the trend to more and more sickness that costs more and more to treat. The root causes of our current crisis are two fold. One, our food, just as it comes off the farm, is getting ever worse. This is not even recognized as a problem. After we process it for an industrial food distribution system, much nutrition is lost too. This is barely recognized as a problem. Until we are better nourished, we will be ever sicker and each generation will become a degeneration. Secondly, our society is suffering from all the evils of monopoly medicine. This is barely recognized. The AMA has a stranglehold on the sick. There is no effective competition for its methods. Alternatives are suppressed. In my version of a better world, if anyone that wanted to could hang out a shingle and offer to diagnose, treat and cure disease, a few quacks would really hurt a few people. But many genuine therapies would appear and the public would be exposed to workable alternatives. If anyone that wanted to market it could put a label on a bottle of pills, power or tincture that said its contents would heal or cure disease, yes, a few people would be poisoned. And a few would die needlessly by failing to get the right treatment. But on the positive side, all this liberty would result in countless new therapies being rediscovered and many new uses for existing substances would appear.

Fundamentally, this is the issue of liberty. I believe it is better to allow choice and options, to permit the dangers that go with liberty to exist. And to allow unfortunate outcomes to occur without intervention into individual lack of intelligence and irresponsibilities. The opposite is our current path–an attempt to regulate and control away all dangers. But this overcontrol results in institutionalized violence and cruelty, inefficiency that is not checked or exposed by the bright light of a better way. As Churchill said, 'democracy is the worst form of government there is–except for all the others.' What he meant is that we must accept that this is an imperfect world. The best this planet can be is when it is at its freest, when restrictions are minimized and when people are allowed to make their own choices, be responsible for their own outcomes and experience the consequences of their own stupidities.

Appendix

Pulse Testing For Allergies

Coca's Pulse Tests are extraordinarily useful and simple tools for at-home allergy detection. My clients have succeeded at using this approach without supervision. Coca's test works on this simple principle: pulse elevations are caused by any allergic reaction. If you know what your normal range of pulse rates are, you can isolate an offending food or substance and eliminate it. Success with Coca's Pulse Test requires only motivation and a little perseverance, because in order to test for food allergies, the diet must be restricted for a few days and your pulse must be accurately taken at specific intervals during the testing period.

The test is based on measurement of the resting pulse rate, something most people have no difficulty learning how to do. The resting rate is how fast the heart beats after a person has been sitting still, comfortably relaxing for three to five minutes. When a person is active the heart beats faster than the resting rate. One measure of aerobic fitness is how quickly the heart is able to return to its resting rate. Well-trained athletes' hearts can adjust from working very hard to a resting rate in only a minute or so; those who are deconditioned can take three to five minutes for their heart to slow from even mild exertion to its stable, resting pace. Those who cannot readily find their own pulse on their wrist or throat can inexpensively purchase a digital watch that gives a pulse reading; this kind of watch is used by athletes to make sure their training pulse is in an acceptable range.

Preparatory to doing Coca's Pulse Test it is necessary to as much as possible eliminate allergic food reactions. This requires the application of discipline for a few days before testing begins. Allergic reactions can go on for several days after a food has been eaten and if you are having a reaction to something eaten many hours or several days previously, it may obscure a reaction to a food just eaten.

1. Stop smoking entirely for at least five days before you do a cigarette test; allergies to cigarettes can take five days to clear. Besides, you shouldn't smoke, anyway!

2. For the first three days, count your resting pulse immediately after awakening in the morning (for one entire minute), and record the reading.

3. During the first three days, take your resting pulse half an hour and again one hour after each meal. It if has elevated more than 12 beats above the resting rate you found upon arising that morning, you may assume that some food at the meal you just ate was an allergen. Temporarily, eliminate from your diet all the foods eaten at the previous meal until you can check them one-by-one a few days later. At the end of these

first three days you may not have many foods left that you can eat. That is okay and to be expected; it is time to begin adding foods back to the diet.

4. Most people who are allergic to foods are allergic to one or more of the following: corn, wheat, milk and cheese, yogurt, meat, alcohol, tobacco. It would be very wise to eliminate these foods too for the first three days, until they are tested.

After three days on this regimen, you can assume that many of your usual allergic food reactions have ceased or at least diminished significantly and that you probably can get reasonably accurate testing results on individual foods. A good indicator of having problems with food allergies in general can also show up during these initial days. If you have eliminated a large number of foods and your resting pulse upon awakening has slowed down by several beats, you can assume you are allergic to foods you were eating.

I would not be at all surprised that by the end of the third day you were only eating a very few fruits and vegetables and had eliminated everything else. A more effective variant of the testing procedure calls for a three or four day water fast to clear all allergies with absolute certainty, and then to introduce foods one at a time as described below.

On the fourth and subsequent few days, take your resting pulse upon arising and then eat a modest quantity of a single food: for example, eat a slice of bread, or a medium sized glass of milk, or an orange, or two tablespoons sugar in dissolved in water, or a few dried prunes, or a peach, or an egg, or a medium-sized potato, or a cup of black coffee without sweetener, or a few ounces of meat, or a stick of celery, or half a cup of raw cabbage, or an onion, or a date, or a few hazelnuts, etc. Count the pulse one half hour later and again one hour after eating the test item.

If any food raises the resting pulse over 12 beats per minute above your morning resting pulse, that food should be eliminated; you are certainly allergic to it or can't digest that much of it. If your pulse has not returned to its morning resting rate one hour later, you are still having an allergic reaction to the food you ate previously and cannot get a decent result on another food until either your pulse slows again or until the next morning. You may, however, continue to eat other foods that you know do not provoke allergic reactions. Because reactions to a food may not clear for many hours, it is wise to eat only small quantities of individual foods if you wish to test many of them in a single day. If a food causes no acceleration of pulse (at least 6 beats above your estimated normal maximal) that food can be tentatively labeled non-allergenic.

After a few days of testing one food an hour, you will become weary of the routine and wish to eat more normally. It may also occur that you cannot test more than one or two foods a day from the very first day because allergic reactions do not clear quickly enough. No problem, the testing period can go on at a lower level of intensity for many weeks, trying one new food each morning upon arising. As you eliminate allergens from your diet one by one, your resting pulse should drop somewhat and it should be easier to discern allergic reactions. After you have worked through all the items in your normal dietary, it would be wise to retest the foods a second time, breaking your fast with one different test item each morning. This second testing round may reveal a few more allergic reactions that were obscured by other allergic reactions the first time through.

Bibliography

Airola, P. N. D., PhD (1974). *How to Get Well*. Phoenix: Health Plus Publishers.

Albrecht, W. A. (1975). *The Albrecht Papers*. Kansas City: Acres, USA.

Alexander, J. (1990). *Blatant Raw Foodist Propaganda!* Nevada City, California: Blue Dolphin Publishing, Inc.

Alsleben, Rudolph H. and Shute, Wilfred E. (1973). *How to Survive the New Health Catastrophes*. Anaheim, CA: Survival Publications.

de Bairacli Levy, Juliette. (1953) *The Complete Herbal Handbook for The Dog and Cat*. London: Faber and Faber.

de Bairacli Levy, Juliette. (1954) *The Complete Herbal Handbook for Farm and Stable*. London: Faber and Faber.

Bieler, H. G., M.D. (1965). *Food Is Your Best Medicine*. New York: Random House. Also Bantam paperback.

Bliznakov, Emile G., M.D. and Hunt, Gerald L. (1987) *The Miracle Nutrient: Coenzyme Q-10*. New York: Bantam Books.

Carrel, A. (1939). *Man the Unknown*. London.

Carrington, H. (1963). *Vitality, Fasting and Nutrition* (reprint of original ca. 1900 edition). Mokelumne Hill, California: Health Research.

Clark, J. (1957). *Hunza: Lost Kingdom of the Himalayas*. London: Hutchinson.

Coca, Arthur F., M.D. (1956) *The Pulse Test: Easy Allergy Detection*. New York: Lyle Stuart, Inc. (Also 1978 paperback edition. New York: Arco Publishing Co.)

Cornaro, L. (1566). Discourses on the Sober Life (reprint: has been through many reprintings by various publishers). Mokelumne Hill, California: Health Research.

Densmore, E. M. D. (1892). How Nature Cures (Reprinted 1976 by Health Research, Mokelumne Hill, California). New York: Stillman & Co.

DeVries, A. (1963). *Therapeutic Fasting*. Greene, Iowa: Chandler Book Co.

Garten, M.O., D.C. (1958) *The Dynamics of Vibrant Health*. Dulzura, CA: Author.

Gerson, M., M.D. (1958). *A Cancer Therapy: Results of Fifty Cases*. DelMar, California: Totality Books.

Gray, R. (1980). *The Colon Health Handbook*. Oakland, California: Rockridge Publishing Company.

Hazzard, L. B. D. O. (1927). *Scientific Fasting: The Ancient and Modern Key to Health* (also Mokelume Hill reprint of original). New York: Grant Publications.

Hawking, David and Pauling, Linus, editors. (1973) *Orthomolecular Psychiatry: Treatment of Schizophrenia*. San Francisco: W. H. Freeman and Company.

Hoffer, Abram and Walker, Morton. (1978) *Orthomolecular Nutrition: New Lifestyle for Super Good Health*. New Cannan: Keats Publishing.

Hopkins, D. P. (1948). *Chemicals, Humus and the Soil*. Brooklyn, NY: Chemical Publishing Company.

Jensen, B. D. C., N.D. *You Can Master Disease*. Solana Beach, California: Bernard Jensen Publishing.

Jensen, B. D. C., & Bell, S. (1981) *Tissue Cleansing Through Bowel Management*. Escondido, California: Bernard Jensen.

Jensen, D. B., D.C. (1976). *Doctor-Patient Handbook*. Provo, Utah: Bi-Worldl Publishers Inc.

Jensen, D. B.and Anderson, Mark (1990). *Empty Harvest: Understanding the link between our food, our immunity and our planet.* Garden City Park, NY: Avery Publishing Group.

Jensen, Bernard and Bodeen, Donald V. (1992) *Visions of Health: Understanding Iridology.* Garden City Park, NY: Avery Publishing Group.

Keys, Ancel, Josef Brozek, Austin Henchel, Olaf Mickelsen and Henry L. Taylor. (1950) *The Biology of Human Starvation.* Two Vols. Minneapolis: University of Minnesota Press.

Kulvinskas, Viktoras.(1972) *Love Your Body.* Wethersfield, Conn: OMango Press.

Kulvinskas, Viktoras. (1975) *Survival Into The 21st Century: Planetary Healers Manual.* Wethersfield, Conn: OMango Press.

Lee, R. *Assorted Lectures: 1923-1963.* Palmyra, WI: Lee Foundation for Nutritional Research.

Lee, R. *Lectures on Malnutrition.* Selene River Press, Fort Collins, CO.

McCarrison, S. R. (1921). *Studies in Deficiency Diseases.* London: Henry Frowde and Hodder & Stoughton. Also Oxford Medical Publications, 1921.

McCarrison, S. R. (1936). "Nutrition and National Health." *Journal of the Royal Society of Arts,* lxxxiv, 1047, 1067, 1087.

McCarrison, S. R. (1982). *Nutrition and Health: being the Cantor Lectures delivered before The Royal Society of Arts 1936 together with two earlier essays.* London: The McCarrison Society.

Natenberg, M. (1957). *The Legacy of Doctor Wylie: and the Administration of His Food and Drug Act.* Chicago: Regent House.

Oswald, J. A. (1989). *Yours for Health: The Life and Times of Herbert M. Shelton.* Franklin, Wisconsin: Franklin Books.

Page, Melvin E. D.D.S. and Abrams, Leon. *Your Body Is Your Best Doctor.* New Cannan: Keats Publishing.

Pearson, Durk and Shaw, Sandy. (1983) *Life Extension: A Practical Scientific Approach.* New York: Warner, 1983.

Pearson, R. B. (1921). *Fasting and Man's Correct Diet* (Reprint, Health Research, Mokelumne Hill, California): originally published by author.

Picton, D. L. J. (1949). *Nutrition and the Soil: Thoughts on Feeding.* New York: Devin-Adair.

Pottenger, F. M. J., M.D (1983). *Pottenger's Cats.* La Mesa, California: Price-Pottenger Nutritional Foundation.

Price, W. A. (1970). *Nutrition and Physical Degeneration.* La Mesa, California: Price-Pottenger Nutrition Foundation.

Quigley, D. T. (1943). *The National Malnutrition.* Palmyra, WI: Lee Foundation for Nutritional Research.

Rodale, J. I. (1949). *The Healthy Hunzas.* Emmaus, PA: Rodale Press.

Shaw, George B. *Back To Methusela.* A play available in many editions.

Schuphan, W. (1965). **Nutritional Values in Crops and Plants**. London: Faber and Faber.

Shelton, H. M. *Health for All* (reprint of original, original date unknown). Mokelumne Hill, California: Health Research.

Shelton, H. M. (1934). *Fasting and Sunbathing.* San Antonio: Dr. Shelton's Health School.

Shelton, H. M. (1935). *Orthotrophy.* San Antonio, Texas: Dr. Shelton's Health School.

Shelton, H. M. (1946). *Getting Well.* San Antonio, Texas: Dr. Shelton's Health School.

Shelton, H. M. (1951). *Food Combining Made Easy.* San Antonio, Texas: Dr. Shelton's Health School.

Shelton, H. M. (1958). *Human Beauty: Its Culture and Hygiene*. San Antonio: Shelton's Health School.

Shelton, H. M. (1971). *Exercise!* Chicago: Natural Hygiene Press.

Sherton, H. M. (1968). *Natural Hygiene: Man's Pristine Way of Life*. San Antonio, Texas: Shelton's Health School.

Sinclair, H. M. (Ed.). (1953). *The Work of Sir Robert McCarrison*. London: Faber and Faber.

Sinclair, Upton. (1921). *The Fasting Cure* (Health Research Reprint, Mokelumne Hill, California, 1955). Pasedena, California: Originally published by the author.

Taylor, R. (1964). *Hunza Health Secrets for Long Life and Happiness*. New York: Award Books.

Tilden, J. H., M.D. (1912). *Diseases of Women and Easy Childbirth* (Reprinted 1962 by Health Research, Mokelumne Hill, CA). Denver: Smith Books Press.

Tilden, J. H., M.D. (1921). *Appendicitis* (Reprinted by Health Research, Mokelumne Hill, CA, 1976). Denver: John Tilden.

Tilden, J. H., M.D. (1921). *Impaired Health: Its Cause and Cure* (reprint of original ca. 1920). Mokelumne Hill, California: Health Research.

Tilden, J. H., M.D. (1939). *Constipation: A New Reading on the Subject* (Reprinted 1960 by Health Research, Mokelumne Hill, California). Denver, Colorado: John Tilden.

Tilden, J. H., M.D., & Trail, R. T., M.D. (1926). *Toxemia Explained & The True Healing Art* (reprint of two original articles; also available through Health Research). Yorktown, Texas: Life Science.

Voisin, Andre. (1959). *Soil, Grass and Cancer*. New York: Philos. Library.

Voisin, A. (1963). *Grass Tetany*. London: Crosby Lockwood and Son Ltd.

Walford, Roy L. M.D. (1983) *Maximum Lifespan*. New York: Avon, 1983.

Walford, Roy L. M.D. (1986) *The 120-Year Diet: How to Double Your Vital Years.* New York: Simon and Schuster.

Weindruch, Richard and Walford, Roy L. (1989) *The Retardation of Aging and Disease by Dietary Restriction.* Springfield, Illinois: Charles C. Thomas.

Whorton, J. (1974). *Before Silent Spring: Pesticides and Public Health in Pre-DDT America.* Princeton, New Jersey: Princeton University Press.

Wigmore, Ann D.D. (1964) *Why Suffer? The Answer? Wheatgrass God's Manna!* Boston: Hippocrates Health Institute.

Williams, R. J. (1971). *Nutrition Against Disease.* New York: Pitmann.

Williams, R. J. (1975). *Physicians' Handbook of Nutritional Science.* Springfield, Illinois: Charles W. Thomas.

Wrench, G. T., M.D. (1938). *The Wheel of Health* (Reprinted 1960 by the Lee Foundation for Nutritional Research; Reprinted by Bernard Jensen International, Escondido, CA, 1990. ed.). London: C.W. Daniel Company Ltd.

Wylie, H. W. (1915). *Not By Bread Alone: The Principles of Human Nutrition.* New York: Hearst's International Library.

Wylie, H. W. (1929). *The History of a Crime Against the Food Law* (Reproduced by Lee Foundation for Nutritional Research, Milwaukee, 1955 ed.). Washington, D.C.: H. W. Wylie.

Wylie, H. W. (1930). *An Autobiography.* Indianapolis: Bobbs-Merrill.

LaVergne, TN USA
21 October 2010

201744LV00005B/37/P